Migraine
Auras

Selected Other Works by Richard Grossinger

Migraine
Auras

When the Visual World Fails

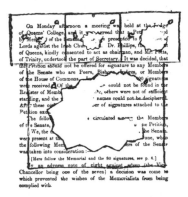

Richard Grossinger

Preface by Klaus Podoll, M.D. and Markus Dahlem, Ph.D.

North Atlantic Books
Berkeley, California

Published by
North Atlantic Books
P.O. Box 12327
Berkeley, California 94712

Cover image by Heather Brady (see p. 20)
Back cover image by Gill Knox
Cover and book design by Paula Morrison

Printed in the United States of America

Migraine Auras: When the Visual World Fails is sponsored by the Society for the Study of Native Arts and Sciences, a nonprofit educational corporation whose goals are to develop an educational and crosscultural perspective linking various scientific, social, and artistic fields; to nurture a holistic view of arts, sciences, humanities, and healing; and to publish and distribute literature on the relationship of mind, body, and nature.

Library of Congress Cataloging-in-Publication Data
Grossinger, Richard, 1944–
    Migraine auras : when the visual world fails / by Richard Grossinger.
        p. ; cm.
    Includes bibliographical references.
    Summary: "This book examines the phenomenon of visual scotomata that is known as migraine aura (whether in tandem with a headache or not); it has intrigued humankind since the dawn of time, yet this is the first book to inform and reassure the many sufferers. With suggestions for healing"—Provided by publisher.
    ISBN-13: 978-1-55643-619-2 (trade paper)
    ISBN-10: 1-55643-619-X (trade paper)
    1. Migraine aura. I. Title.
    [DNLM: 1. Migraine with Aura—complications. 2. Complementary Therapies. 3. Migraine with Aura—therapy. 4. Vision Disorders—etiology. WL 344 G878m 2006]
    RC392.G77 2006
    616.8'4912—dc22

                                        2006009446
1 2 3 4 5 6 7 8 9 UNITED 12 11 10 09 08 07 06

*For John Upledger, Eugene Alexander, Frank Lowen, Robert Zeiger,
and Michael Wagner, healers who have shown me the way*

Table of Contents

Disclaimer

Medical knowledge is ever changing. As new research and clinical experiences broaden our knowledge, changes in treatment and drug therapy may be required. The author and editors of the material herein have consulted sources believed to be reliable in their efforts to provide information that is complete and in accordance with the standards accepted at the time of publication.

However, the author, editors, publisher, or any other party who has been involved in the preparation of this work, do not warrant the information contained herein and are not responsible for any errors or omissions resulting from the use of such information.

Readers are encouraged to confirm the information contained herein with other sources to best suit their particular situations.

This book is offered solely for educational purposes. Therefore, neither the author nor the publisher assumes any responsibility for the use that any reader makes of the information it contains. The reader is simply urged to consider the material presented and to use it at his or her own risk.

Some of the product names, patents, and registered designs referred to in this book are in fact registered trademarks or proprietary names, even though specific reference to this fact is not always made in the text. Therefore, the appearance of a name without designation as proprietary is not to be construed as a representation by the publisher that it is in the public domain.

Preface

By Klaus Podoll, M.D. and Markus Dahlem, Ph.D.

Richard Grossinger's book *Migraine Auras* is a twentieth (or rather twenty-first) century migraine sufferer's personal record and synthesis of what is currently known about this enigmatic phenomenon. Migraine auras may herald the headache of an acute migraine attack or occur without any pain. The seemingly infinite varieties of aura portrayed in this book consist of brief interruptions of everyday life consciousness, occurring to people of all ages at unpredictable times, from Hildegard of Bingen to Marvin Minsky. These episodes are described by them as visions of hell or, alternately, glimpses of heaven.

Grossinger, who has a Ph.D. in anthropology, has forty years experience as a writer and ethnographer, his previous work ranging from experimental literary prose and oral history to popular science on medicine, cosmology, and embryology. In *Migraine Auras*, amalgamating motifs of his earlier books, he draws on autobiographical experiences; accounts from doctors, friends, and casual acquaintances; literature (both medical and fictional); fine arts; and post-Gutenberg media like films, CDs, and, last but not least, the Internet which is here mined for the first time as a source of original data in a monograph on the phenomenon in question.

That this is a book from a non-medical writer accounts for both its strengths and limits. For instance, it is not primarily an evidence-based scientific account but includes methodologically deviant speculation in the traditions of psychoanalysis, the Jacksonian principle of evolution and dissolution of the nervous system, and homeopathy. That also turns out to be one of its virtues, as it provides migraine sufferers with new ways to imagine and experience their auras. The author invites the reader on a journey exploring the phantasmagoria of a psychoneural experience that is usually weird, traumatic, and stigmatized as well as beautiful, revelatory, and consciousness-expanding. Beyond the scope of books akin to *What You Always Wanted to Ask Your Doctor But Didn't*, Grossinger raises questions and provides answers vis a vis those aspects of the migraine aura experience that are excluded from the common medical discourse: its ontological, semeiological, and psychospiritual dimensions. He thus offers his readers and fellow "sufferers" the outlines of a "migraine-aura aesthetics" that can serve as a valuable means to cope with this human—all-too-human—condition as a gift rather than an illness.

—Klaus Podoll, M.D., Clinic for Psychiatry and Psychotherapy, University Hospital Aachen, Aachen, Germany

—Markus Dahlem, Ph.D., Clinic for Neurology II, Medical Faculty, Otto-von-Guericke University Magdeburg, Magdeburg, Germany

I.
The Nature and Experience of Migraine Auras

Introduction

Suddenly motorists are unable to see the road ahead of them, a portion of it disappearing into a flashing spot; yet most keep on driving. A pilot with a 747 full of passengers confronts a splotched, roiling runway; yet he gets the plane smoothly onto the ground and doesn't report the incident. If he did, he might lose his job.

Men and women at conferences watch the auditorium turn into a cubist painting in which they cannot recognize their colleagues; yet they persist in their participation, even addressing the group, without confessing. Doctors continue examining patients; factory workers persevere at their machines; actors remain in character.

Athletes may leave contests because of auras. The public is told that a player has a migraine and will not return, but this gives the misleading impression of an incapacitating headache rather than a distortion of sight. When Kareem Abdul-Jabbar (in the 1990s) or Steve Francis (a decade later) had to skip the second half of a basketball game, the assumption was that both were experiencing head pain, not that they couldn't see a hoop to shoot at.

The word "migraine" has inexplicably become a smokescreen behind which to hide migraine auras, which are very different experiences and can occur without headaches.

Ocular auras are sudden, seemingly causeless and sourceless disturbances of sight in the brain—not the eyes—and they result in anomalies of vision, often extraordinarily bright patterns, intrusive shapes, and blind spots. Lasting at least four minutes but usually less than an hour, these fully reversible neuropsychological hallucinations are often characterized by disorientation and mild aphasia.

If one did not know that they were experiencing a relatively benign, transient phenomenon, they might think that they had a dire pathology.

In ordinary discourse migraines are pulsating, throbbing headaches with one-sided pangs, different from sinus and tension headaches or headaches arising from other causes. American artist Janet McKenzie writes: "Mine come in blinding strokes of pain, in two or three beats of pain, in one spot. They feel like lightning that has gotten trapped inside my head and is trying to flash or burn its way out."[1]

A British patient offered comparable forensics: "No two attacks are alike of course—sometimes the pain is like a tight band across the head, producing a general sort of ache, whereas other times I feel as if a spade blade of intense pain from above my eyes was cutting through to the back of my head, from where it sends shafts of pain downward to the base of my skull.

"Quite often there is a pain at the back of my neck where the muscles seem to be all tensed up, although on many occasions the main discomfort is concentrated just above and below my right eye."[2]

These attacks are one guise of migraine.

The word "migraine" derives from the Middle English *mygrame* and French *megrim,* turning into *migraine* with a misreading of "in" for "m": a name for a form of "headache." Yet the terms "migraine" and "super-headache" are by no means synonymous. A headache is neither a sole nor necessary nor even primary criterion of a migraine; it is at most its acme or trademark. A German writer, Erich Kæstner summarizes this misnomer in a *double entendre:* "Migraines are headaches, even if you don't have any."[3]

In medical parlance a migraine *can be* a headache, but it can also be nausea, diarrhea, an ephemeral psychosis, or an aura—or all of these *with or without a headache.* "Migraine" is a loose confederation of altered neurological and psychosomatic states within a single biophysical matrix.

Traditional "migraine" terminology makes further distinctions: So-called "common migraines" are aura-less pulsing unilateral headaches. "Classical" migraines, by contrast, are headaches with auras.

A classical migraine comprises an aura followed by a headache that usually begins as the aura is dissipating. It is called "classical" because of the affiliation of auras with headaches in the recent annals of migraine. Spontaneous visual distortions have been described throughout history, but the association of a class of them with migraines was not recognized until the late nineteenth century.

Auras are considered forerunners and accompanists of headaches, either their prodome or incipient phase. "The pain which follows is on the side on which the central function is distributed, that is, on the side of the head opposite to that to which the visual sensations are objectively referred. If these seem to occupy the left side of the field of vision the pain usually begins on the right side of the head."[4]

Migraine headaches without visual accompaniment are called "common" because auras are deemed exceptions or adjuncts to cephalgia and are now known to occur independently of it.

Today people mostly skip the old terminology and refer to "migraine with aura" or "migraine without aura."

Current estimates are that approximately 15 percent of migraine-headache sufferers experience an initiating aura. About 10 percent of auras precede their headaches by anywhere from a few seconds to an hour (but usually at least five minutes). The rest overlap with them to one degree or another. Classical auras vary in length but generally fall into the half-hour range, though the ensuing headaches may last up to twelve hours or—very rarely—longer. In a rare migraine complication, called persistent aura (formerly labeled migraine aura status), the aura may even last longer than a week!

"Auras without headaches," technically "acephalgic migraines," are sometimes called "migraine equivalents" (see p. 114) and may be identified by the acronym MAWOH (migraine aura without headache).

About 20 percent of all migraineurs report auras without headaches at some time or other, and at least 3 percent of migraineurs *only* experience auras, never headaches.[5] But so many people likely suffer from headacheless auras without documenting them that the combined incidence of classical migraines and MAWOHs probably makes them *more common* than common migraines.

The fact that ocular auras can arise without headaches contributes to their routine misidentification as well as the consternation that can accompany a first attack. If a headache occurred at the same time or soon thereafter, the person would likely correlate the visual distortion with the pain and *know* what was happening to him: a migraine discharging across sensory boundaries. In the absence of pain, the "silent" moving artifact is stunning and inexplicable.

Now here is a further twist: A migraine aura is often visual but may also be a numbness pattern or some other altered sensation. Auras can affect just about any neural pathway—again either with or without a visual component and with or without a headache.

Visual distortions are the most common auras; yet auras comprise symptoms as diverse as tingling, muscular or motor weakness, hemiplegia (paralysis on one side of the body), faintness, decreased levels of consciousness, impediments of language formation and memory, lethargy, sleepiness, spasms (almost anywhere), unpleasant temperature variations (surges of heat or cold or both simultaneously), and other spontaneous sensations, as well as disturbances of taste (food eaten during the migraine does not taste like itself), hearing (tinnitus, buzzing), tactility (prickling or crawling sensations, the latter known as formication), kinesthesia (dizziness, loss of balance and/or sense of direction), and strange or wrong smells without a source (something may also smell distinctly like something else). All of these are homologous to the more familiar visual aura.

Twinkling, flickering, and scintillating effects that accompany both tactile and visual auras are known as *choreas*—jerky, involuntary movements, often of the face and extremities. They also characterize other diseases of the nervous system.

While this book deals with migraines as well as their auras, its concentration is on visual (or ocular) auras. However, in many instances, what I will say about those applies to other auras and migraine headaches too.

My objective is to describe and explain migraine auras and to offer support to sufferers. I will archive wide-ranging descriptions of people's auras; discuss their possible relationships to other physical, psychosomatic, and psychospiritual conditions; interpret their causes and meaning; distinguish them from other, often more serious pathologies; survey the present state of migraine research; and review the range of treatment options and their relative pros and cons. Because there is no *bona fide* cure or preventive medicine for migraines or auras, relief must come mainly in the form of holistic integration and deeper understanding.

Although it is justifiable to regard migraines as waking nightmares or "bad trips" and wish them to go away, a "victim" could also turn them into a rich experience by appreciating how our brain and psyche collaborate. Not only are interruptions of ordinary perception normal, but they may serve important functions.

Testimony

"I have frequently experienced a sudden failure of sight. The general sight did not appear affected; but when I looked at any particular object, it seemed as if something brown, and more or less opaque, was interposed between my eyes and it, so that I saw it indistinctly, or sometimes not at all...." So begins a nineteenth-century account of a migraine aura.

"After it had continued a few moments, the upper or lower edge appeared bounded by an edging of light of a zigzag shape, and coruscating nearly at right angles to its length. The coruscation always appeared to be in one eye; but both it and the cloud existed equally whether I looked at an object with one or both eyes open.... The cloud and the coruscation ... would remain from twenty minutes, sometimes to half an hour.... They were in me never followed by headache ... [but] generally went off with a movement in the stomach producing eructation."[6]

Hubert Airy's aura narrative from 1870 remains one of the most precise and complete:

"[A] small angled sphere suddenly appears in one side of the combined field.... [I]t rapidly enlarges, first as a circular zigzag, but on the inner side, towards the medial line, the regular outline becomes faint, and, as the increase in size goes on, the outline here becomes broken, the gap becoming larger as the whole increases, and the original circular outline becomes oval. The form assumed is roughly concentric with the edge of the field of vision.... [T]he lines which constitute the outline meet at right angles or larger angles.... When this angled oval has extended through the greater part of the half-field the upper portion expands; it seems to overcome at last some resistance in the immediate neighborhood of the fixing point ... so that a bulge occurs in the part above, and the angular elements of the outline here enlarge.... After this final stage occurs, the outer lower part of the outline disappears. The final expansion near the centre progresses with great rapidity, and ends in a whirling centre of light from which sprays of light seem flying off."[7]

An 1895 paper reports a woman who, after looking at a brilliant light, would see a vista of bright stars. "One of the stars, brighter than the rest, would start from the right lower corner of the field of vision, and pass across the field, generally quickly, in a second, sometimes more slowly, and when it reached the left side would break up and leave a blue area in which luminous points were moving."[8]

In a 1904 account from the same author, a man named Beck was taking his seat at a family dinner when a "zig-zag spectrum, coloured red and blue, suddenly appeared, surrounding the edge of the plate before him." He was startled by this luminous pulsation that was neither decoration nor food: "As I looked curious my wife said, 'Why do you not carve?' On taking my eyes off the plate I said to them, 'The zig-zag rainbow colours are gone out of the window.'"[9] That is, they left the table and followed his visual field. This is a description of a pericentral aura (see Figure 7 for a comparable motif).

A more recent, clinical record succinctly authenticates these historical protocols: "The disturbance which occurs approximately every six months reportedly begins centrally as a small, bilateral, circular distortion, and then expands, over a twenty-minute period, into an enlarging three-quarter circle of brightly colored and flickering lights described as being 'similar to multiple small prisms laid side-by-side in semicircular fashion.' The disturbance continues to enlarge until it grows out of the patient's field of vision."[10]

My own first experience of a migraine aura came at age forty-eight without forewarning. While absorbed in the morning newspaper, I suddenly had trouble understanding a sentence. I was unsure what the problem was. It seemed as though the mechanism of reading and comprehension had broken down. I tried adjusting my head, as though the light was wrong (either too bright or too faint), but that didn't help. I moved the paper closer and then further away, imagining that it had gotten out of focus. I still couldn't read it, and I couldn't understand why. I also could no longer comprehend the article. I began to get frantic.

Then it occurred to me that the difficulty lay on the page. It was badly printed. There was a smudge over one of the letters such that it was indecipherable; it no longer looked like a familiar typographical letter but a hieroglyph, something that might be found on a wall in a Mayan ruin. Perhaps dirt had gotten on the press. But then why should one misprinted letter make an entire page illegible?

All at once, to my dismay I realized that other letters were turning hieroglyphic and, as I moved my eyes over the page, different ones were being replaced by characters becoming glyphs. The distortion was in *me*. Even as I was comprehending this terrible thing, letters and then whole words began to disappear.

When an aura arises while one is reading, the initiating event is somewhat like a piece of mottled glass suddenly placed over a part of the page. The flaw starts out tiny, about pinhead size, but grows until it becomes a spreading moil, a mirage reliable enough to have a scientific name. It is called a *scotoma* (the plural is *scotomata*). The term *scintillating scotoma* is used to designate its peculiar luminous pulsation. This greedy shape covers or erases text and scenery, gradually swelling and evolving through a variety of different oscillating patterns before dissipating while traveling, usually in one or the other lateral direction, out of the field of vision. The following description from a 1971 scientific article is typical:

"The ... disturbance ... begins near the center of the visual field as a small gray area with indefinite boundaries. If this area first appears during reading, as it often does, then the migraine is first noticed when words are lost in a region of 'shaded darkness.' Dur-

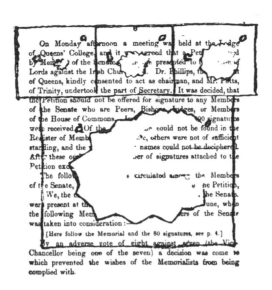

Figure 1: Representation by astronomer Hubert Airy of the development of a migraine aura over his newspaper. The luminous zigzag is represented by the black line. (From William Richard Gowers, *Subjective Sensations of Sight and Sound,* Philadelphia: P. K. Blakiston's Son & Co., 1904, p. 26.)

ing the next few minutes the gray area slowly expands into a horseshoe with bright zigzag lines appearing at the expanding outer edge. The lines are small at first and grow as the blind area expands and moves outward toward the periphery of the visual field."[11]

Scotoma, the Classical Greek word for "dizziness," describes the hallucination over the visual field. It trails a blind spot, the so-called *negative scotoma,* in which nothing can be seen.

Everywhere the scotoma does not occupy is usually more or less normal landscape. "The loss of sight, in the form of the expanding spectrum, is always within the angled oval. Outside the limiting line, vision is preserved; within it, vision is lost; at first over the whole area; afterwards, when the sphere is broken and has become oval, the loss is most intense close to the limiting line and becomes less towards the middle,"[12] as is shown in Figure 1.

A scotoma is a replacement of vision—not in the eye, which still receives appropriate streams of information through the lens and retina and dispatches them faithfully into the optic nerves—but in the ocular aspect of the cerebral cortex and/or the cerebral field where the visual signal registers and is processed. The brain no longer integrates optic impulses in the ordinary way but instead imposes its own intrinsic excitation converted into a shape or erasure that has little to do with its actual functioning or psychological and cultural role as a brain.

Unlike many other visual disturbances, a migraine aura cannot be halted or alleviated by movement of the head or eyes, by closing the eyes, or even by going to sleep—the lambent flame on Beck's dinner plate is standard. One sufferer notes: "The actual effect follows wherever I look (I can't escape it by looking around)."[13] This indelible quality is because the artifact is in the brain. It appears in both eyes simultaneously, unabated when the eyes are closed, except that it changes from a distortion into a flashing geometry.

After my first encounter with a migraine aura, an experience similar to the "deteriorating" newspaper recurred every few months. A blank spot or mottle appeared somewhere in my view (for instance, on a wall, within an object, or against the sky), as though I were looking through a window with a bleb in it. The mottle proceeded to transit the visual field, growing and changing into zigzags and multiform shapes before exploding into dizzying smoke and then dissolving, leaving a hangover of gradually diminishing oscillation and distortion. The patch originated at different sites, never dead center but toward the right or the left of the visual field; it always moved toward its closer border. With my eyes open, it was a dark and crinkled disfiguration; with them closed, it became a scintillating light.

The second time this happened I went to an ophthalmologist

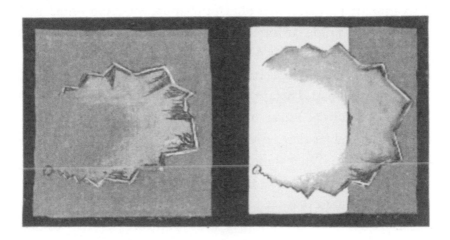

Figure 2: Dr. Airy's transposition of the aura in Figure 1 when the viewer faces (left) a dark background and (right) a bright window. (From William Richard Gowers, *Subjective Sensations of Sight and Sound,* Philadelphia: P. K. Blakiston's Son & Co., 1904, p. 27.)

who, after an exam with instruments, reported that he found nothing in my dilated eyes corresponding to what I had described. A few floaters perhaps . . . that was it. Of course, the aura had long passed by then; yet I found it hard to believe that so dramatic an event left no scar, nary a fingerprint.

I did not pursue the matter. The episode dropped out of my immediate awareness into vague concern.

Each time during an attack I was anxious and agitated but, when my vision cleared after a half hour or so, I went on with my life. I didn't know what "it" was. It bewildered me that the distortion persisted when my eyes were closed and appeared identically in both eyes. Even though it seemed to cure itself, I didn't have a good feeling about it. It looked too much like a universal warning sign.

Only after the visual disruption had occurred maybe four or five times over a year did I get an opportunity to recount it to a doctor during a routine exam. I expected him to attend closely. Instead, he seemed matter-of-fact—he guessed that I was having migraines. While pleased by the harmless diagnosis, I worried that these things didn't seem like migraines. Of course, I was thinking "headaches" and "pain," as most people initially do.

The symptoms did not get progressively worse; displays remained infrequent and brief and always ended without consequences, leaving things much as they were before. Over the next several years I became reassured that these defects were neither sight- nor life-threatening. As my eyes were becoming more myopic anyway with aging, I attributed them to some trait of overall blurrier vision. I had had excellent eyesight throughout youth, and my supposition was that I was out of the loop on the sorts of exotic aberrations that can obtrude as people's vision weakens. I had also been experiencing a strange occasional flickering in my eyes for a year or so, and I considered that these new deficits were a more elaborate version of the same thing (see p. 72).

Yet I also recalled vague rumors from long ago, perhaps in a movie. No matter how much I reassured myself, when these shapes occurred, there was a menacing, macabre quality to them, like science-fiction landscapes of uninhabitable planets or condensed, obliterated narratives of terrible deeds committed in ancient times or other dimensions. I tried to make my existence invisible to these trespassers, to get them to ignore me. Alternately I proclaimed them innocent moiré effects of worsening sight.

On two occasions when a figment occurred while I was driving alone, I concentrated on the road, moving my head as I needed to, and managed to get to my destination without mishap. Another time I parked on the shoulder and switched places with my wife.

Three years after the first aura, a psychotherapist whom I was seeing told me that he had attended a conference the previous weekend and the condition I described had been categorized to a "t" by one of the speakers. It was called a "migraine without headache." He was confident of the match.

That reassured me more than the M.D.'s assessment because I trusted that the therapist listened to my exact words and analyzed them at more than one level. Still I didn't believe he grasped exactly what I was witnessing. I assumed that he had heard an account of something enough *like* my "thing" to sound the same, but not as weird or portentous.

I went ten more years with chronic ocular auras, maybe fifteen a year at the max (though some twelve-month periods with none), using "migraine" as my probationary explanation. During the procession I would be mildly to acutely alarmed but, as long as it followed an established protocol, I marked and counted off each stage, while impatiently awaiting the finale. I would be quite upset, even terrified, by the slightest variation from the "norm," as this was a rabid wolf that needed to be given a wide berth and kept on its fixed course. When the world returned to normal, I breathed my sigh of relief.

Then, during a period of two weeks in April and May of 2004, I experienced a cluster of scotomata. The onslaught consisted of three pairs of brilliant, pulsating auras, six altogether over ten days, the second in each pair occurring within eighteen hours of the first. It was as though I were the target of moving crop circles transmitting an alien equation. Each episode in a pair was intrinsically related to the other, completing its pattern. If the first began with a conventional blind spot dilating into flashing zigzags, the second manifested as full-blown zigzags and then generated a blind spot. If the first scotoma exited to the left, the second exited to the right.

My fears about these intruders climaxed; they lurked like poisonous spiders, epileptic robots about to explode into some lethal pathology—they certainly weren't just migraines. In addition, a friend had just been diagnosed with a brain tumor after undergoing spontaneous visual deformations.

At the sixth in the cluster, I jettisoned what remained of my composure, dashed to the computer—scotoma blocking the screen—found my way to the Alta Vista site, and typed in a daringly candid "advanced search"—bring what it might—listing as "any of the above": "zigzag," "blind spot," "dot," "flash," "kaleidoscope," etc. To my astonishment (and elation), the word "migraine" sprouted everywhere like mushrooms after rain. Both the doctor and therapist were right. There *was* such a thing as a "migraine without headache."

I chose a chatroom (www.halfbakery.com) entitled "Migraine Visual Aura Simulation"; here was precisely the strange sequence I was experiencing, presented again and again with variations. A woman named Sarenka wrote:

"I am one of the unlucky many who experience classic migraines, which are always preceded by a visual aura. What does this aura look like? Mine tend to fit the usual descriptions: flashing, zigzag patterns, blinding an area in my field of vision. I read that the exact effect is different from person to person, but for me, they tend to start out as a small, blinding dot that reminds me of what it looks like after accidentally being blinded by a glare or the sun. The dot starts to flash and grow over the next half hour to hour, resembling a C, a backwards C, a sideways V, or even an oval or complete circle. The pattern tends to be off-center as it grows and gradually moves to the outer edges of my field of vision. [It] looks to me like a distinct flashing chain of connected triangles."[14]

In another entry she remarked: "When auras occur, it's like a blind spot, but with the crazy movement of the classic zigzagged C-shape thingy. This makes it hard to see and is also distracting and uncomfortable to me.... I used to only get the growing C-shaped auras on the right side and, if a headache followed, it was always on the left side of my head.... I used not to get the headaches at all at first and even went to get my eyes checked, where I first heard the

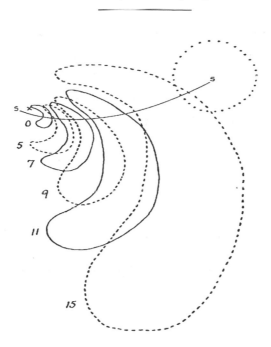

Figure 3: Contours of a scintillating scotoma mapped at intervals of zero, five, seven, nine, eleven, and fifteen minutes. Scintillations occurred solely in the region above the line *s-s*. (From Karl Spencer Lashley, "Patterns of Cerebral Integration Indicated by Scotomas of Migraine," *Archives of Neurological Psychiatry,* 1941, Vol. 46, p. 333.)

diagnosis 'ocular migraines.' They now occur more frequently, on either the left or right, and are usually followed by a headache, which is always on the opposite side."[15]

A contributor named Squeak corroborated: "Mine start as a flashing, pulsating C that grows and flips until I can't see."[16]

Karl Spencer Lashley's 1941 account could well belong on the forum: "The scotoma [usually] starts as a disturbance of vision ... a small blind or scintillating spot, subtending less than 1 degree, in or immediately adjacent to the foveal field. This spot rapidly increases in size and drifts away from the fovea toward the temporal field of one side. Usually both quadrants of one side only are involved, the right and the left being affected with about equal frequency. Occasionally the scotoma is confined to one quadrant.... [T]he disturbance of vision ... is limited to the neighborhood of the macula and spreads rapidly toward the temporal field. With increase in size the disturbed area moves or 'drifts' across the visual field, so that its central margin withdraws from the macular region as its peripheral margin invades the temporal...."[17]

Bristolz, another contributor, offers these musings: "I, too, am a classic migraine sufferer (or was, they seem to have disappeared in the last two years and neither me nor my doctors can figure out what changed or why—not that I'm complaining or anything). For me, zigzag patterns in blue and yellow; a horizontal line that cuts my field-of-vision in half and makes the top part out of register with the bottom; a sense that there is smoke in the air and the crescent-shaped thingy that looks like it's composed of little cascading bars are all part of the visual phenomenon. Also, I get the sensation that there is a wind on my face. If it weren't for the nausea and oh-my-gawd pain, it might be kind of fun."[18]

The smoke that Bristolz reports is a feature familiar to me at the end of most aura sequences. As the flashing zigzags and/or other elements parade off the edge of my field of vision, they don't so much slide seamlessly into unseen territory as come apart with the quality of endless string unraveling, except that the string has a cloudy or smoky texture that causes it to melt and float and pinwheel about, somewhat like a pattern of "seeing stars." Gowers describes "a whirling centre of light from which sprays of light seem flying off."[19] This makes me quite dizzy, paradoxically as the scotoma's motif is no longer visible, yet justifying etymology.

Bristolz concludes by distinguishing MAWOHs from classical migraines, "My father has 'painless migraine' with just weird visual stuff. My mother, on the other hand, would get taken out of service for three days or so. I guess it was destiny for me."[20]

Another website visitor named Mkstar, upon reading that others undergo similar encounters, expresses relief and gratitude similar to my own:

"All I can say is THANK YOU. I thought I was losing my mind. About two months ago I was driving back to work from my lunch break and thought I looked at the sun or something. I was seeing spots and they weren't going away. I was having trouble focusing on the road. I got back to work and looked at myself in the mirror. I felt like I was suddenly tripping on acid or something. I went into my office and said, 'Um, guys, I don't know how to explain this but I am seeing spots. My vision is blurry and I can't seem to focus. Can someone take me home?'

"On my way outside, the 'spots' became larger and larger and moved out to the perimeter of my vision, and then I lost peripheral vision. I simply could not see out of the corner of my eyes!

"I called the doctor and sat in the dark. Then an hour later it happened again, so I analyzed it this time. It started out like a small flash; I describe it now as looking like a 'watermark,' a circle that grew larger and larger, moved out to the visual perimeters, a loss of peripheral vision, and then I noticed a headache. Well, I was worried I was having a stroke, and that just made me more anxious. The doctor said at the time it might be a migraine.... Two months later I had another one. I was at work and, let me tell you, I cannot function when it happens. Mine last for approximately fifteen minutes so far....

"I just want to thank you for putting my mind at ease, although I am still worried about having a stroke. When I read this page, I was like, 'At least I am not the only one with these strange visual experiences!'"[21]

On a different website that invites migraine "live journals," Heather Brady chronicles her first encounter with a scotoma (April, 2004). This aura appears on the cover:

"Marshie and I were just hanging out yesterday when I noticed a tiny spot in my field of vision, almost like a floater. I ignored it until I realized it was getting bigger. It was like the afterimage you get when you look at a bright light for too long, but I had done no such thing, and it continued to grow. I started to freak when I noticed that it was in both eyes, even when closed. By this time it was a large circle that filled most of the window and appeared to have wildly pulsating, colourful borders. I was beside myself with panic.

"Thankfully, level-headed Marshie did a couple of Google searches and we soon determined that I was not having a stroke, but I was still extremely alarmed. A call to Telehealth Ontario advised that the wait time to speak to a nurse was well over an hour...." A few minutes later, after recalling the migraine experience of another poster (named zero gravity), Brady noticed that she was calmer, "and the apparition had gotten so large that it began to dissipate at the edge of my vision, like a cloud passing over the sun. About 10 minutes later, it was gone and the headache hit. Indeed, it was just a migraine. Not a stroke, not a brain tumour, not a detached retina, but a lousy migraine. Scary shit, nonetheless."[22]

Barnzenen similarly feared "a tumor might have formed and started affecting me, or spinal meningitis." His other symptoms included hypersensitivity to light, sound, and touch, "slurred speech, loss of some feeling in the right leg, stiff neck, and pain-induced vomiting." He jokes about his neurologist confirming "that I do have a brain (CAT proved it) and that I'm not dying of anything."[23]

On another website Jim M. writes: "Just found out the other day what the crazy moving sawtooth arc was ... scintillating scotoma! I thought it was something serious for the past 8 years when they started suddenly on a Sunday morning. Went to many eye docs over

the years ... always the same diagnosis 'your eyes are perfectly normal.' I had the idea it was a 'brain job' for a long time because I had
deduced that it was going across both eyes. My vision looks just like
the images on the computer ... no migraine [i.e., no headache] ...
just the flashing, sawtooth lines which form a sideways V or arc and
which get larger and larger until it disappears. Nice to know there are
so many of us. ... bet the eye doctors make a fortune out of this
scary event."[24]

I printed out a batch of these accounts and was reading them a
month later on a flight from Oakland to Seattle when I noticed the
man seated next to me peeking at my pages. As I caught his attention,
he exclaimed, "My god, that's what I get! I never knew what it was."
He asked if he could borrow the printout to show to his wife across
the aisle. I handed it to him, and he carried it to her seat. I watched
her startled acknowledgment. Even more surprising—as soon as
she began perusing it, the man seated next to her began eaves-
dropping. I could overhear him telling her that this was the first
explanation he had ever come across for "those damn light shows."

The "publisher" in me was now alerted. After first ascertaining
that there was no contemporary book on migraine auras, I spent
the next eighteen months gathering the best material from inter-
views, texts, journals, Internet articles, and chatrooms while trying
to hire a technical writer. However, the various freelancers I contacted either found the topic too abstruse and challenging or
requested preposterous sums of money for the job. In addition, it
was clear from their outlines that all of them intended to rehash
material already widely available, i.e., turn out a repetitive book
reorganized from stock material. At that point, I decided to assemble my own improvised notes into a book.

Since I am not an expert on either the etiology of migraines or
neuroscience, this text does not emphasize post-modern microbi-

ology or pharmacology. I cover these topics subjectively, as they tend to offer little in the way of clarification or remedy. With no confirmed explanation or cure for auras, there would not be much of a book without exploring their ontology and phenomenology. Since I didn't want the sort of tedious song-and-dance that appears in most headache guides, I also used "migraine" as a departure for speculations on consciousness, personal identity, and the sensory basis of meaning.

Oliver Sacks' *Migraine*

If one were to try to find a whole book on migraine auras prior to this one, he or she would be disappointed. There are no contemporary, in-print books addressing just visual auras,* though there are innumerable volumes, of course, on migraine headaches and also plenty of textbooks of ophthalmology and neurology that mention visual auras, usually as a prodrome of headaches. Despite the experience of scotomata by so many and their window into the mechanism of the brain, few authors have explored the phenomenon in and of itself.

Neurologist Oliver Sacks' brilliant book *Migraine,* published in 1970 and revised in 1992, is the exception. It is the best source of information on visual auras that I have found. Lucid and thorough, it is recommended reading for anyone who wants to investigate this topic further. Out of 300 pages all told, more than 100 address just auras. Although some parts of his book are a bit outdated from a medical point of view, everything Sacks says about auras is inter-

---

*Limited-edition catalogues of migraine art have been assembled by Sandoz Laboratories and the British Migraine Association, and two titles on migraine philosophy and art have been published under similar auspices (see pp. 50–51).

esting, and I will try to do justice to his considerations, for they are unique in contemporary writing on the subject.

At the same time, I will prioritize visual auras over the larger migraine complex. This is partly for the benefit of those who suffer auras without headaches; partly to understand extreme hallucinations and ocular distortions of diverse sorts, not just migraines; and partly to expand migraine mythology and aesthetics. Although I am interested in the association of auras with cephalgia, my responsibility is the aura, whether it comes with head pain, precedes head pain, or is totally painless.

Opening his 1992 Revised Edition, Sacks attempts to cheer those who have suffered auras: "Many patients ... who experience a migraine aura, or an attack of classical migraine for the first time have no idea what is happening to them, and may be terrified that they have a stroke, a brain tumour, or whatever—or conversely, that they are going mad, or suffering from bizarre hysteria. It is an immense reassurance for such patients to learn that what they have is neither grave nor factitious, but a morally neutral, recurrent yet essentially benign condition which they share with countless others, and which is well understood."[25]

A migraine aura is not a sign of pathology; equally it is not hysteria or insanity; it is an innocent neural discharge.

By "not factitious," I take Sacks to mean that migraines and their auras are not deep-seated or profound but relatively superficial and transient. They are one of a variety of interruptions of "normal" functioning that happen to people of all ages at unpredictable times.

By "morally neutral," I take him to mean that they are neither visions from angels nor punishments for lapses of character, failed hygiene, or bad diet. They are emotional and psychophysiological episodes with their own biochemistry and natural history and probably their own role in the homeostasis of body-mind.

Definition of the Aura and Scotoma

Visual auras can be classified in three phases, though many sufferers do not get to a third tier and, in others, the first and second are so close to each other as to be indistinguishable. This may sometimes indicate that an aura is already in the second stage by the time it is noticed.

The so-called positive (as opposed to vision-deficient) components of the first two phases commence with phosphenes (electric-like sparklings in the visual field, which spread like ripples in a pond), halos, nimbi, and/or fulminations, as well as broader patterns of lights and geometric shapes (red and green or red and yellow triangles or hexagons, objects colored and/or with brilliant outlines, etc.).

The negative components are blind spots and dissociations and disorientations of the visual field.

Phosphenes create the effect of "seeing stars" after falling down. They may also resemble persistent floaters. Writing in the halfbakery chatroom, Malakh describes them as if "someone took a handful of glitter and threw it into the air. A lot of small sparkly things ... fly around."[26] Swarming in the dozens, they dance across the field of vision as embers and/or flashes.*

Airy emphasizes their mobile brilliance: "[It] may be likened to the effect produced by the rapid gyration of small water-beetles as they are seen swarming in a cluster on the surface of the water in sunshine."[27]

A more recent account summarizes a century of reports: "Terms

---

*In European football (American soccer), the act of "heading" a ball can elicit "shooting stars" that turn into phosphenes that then progress to a scotoma during play.

such as 'sparkling, dancing lights,' 'vibrating light,' 'wiggly line,' 'shimmering like heat off a hot road,' 'jagged flashes,' and 'flickering light' are … used to describe [phosphenes'] occurrence. Colors most often reported are red, gold or yellow, green, and blue or purple."[28]

Quite commonly there is only one phosphene. Originating as if an afterglow or blind spot from a bright light, its neural fixation does not fade but develops shape and structure and sometimes color (note the 1895 report on p. 9).

Another migraineur recounts a slightly different permutation: "My visual aura[s] … usually look like sperm … a bright silvery light that swims around in my vision and leaves a little tail behind it."[29] (moved ahead two)

These fluctuations in description indicate differences in neural excitation, personal perception, and use of language, but the variations subtend a central design.

Whether single or multiple and whatever their original manifestation, the initiating light or lights usually complexify into patterns, disks, and simple geometries. Their configuration creates the aura's spectrum and, with its effects, constitutes the scotoma.

The scotoma (with its positive and negative aspects) represents the next phase of organization. In the most prevalent sequence one dot or phosphene, while taking on various shapes, expands and travels toward the margin of the visual field. Often it dilates, like Sarenka's, into a giant crescent or backwards C or "kidney-shaped dazzles"[30] before developing a series of connected zigzags or triangles. The central margin may withdraw from the general pattern while the peripheral margin permeates it, as the initial mote becomes a blemish with "chromatic edgings."[31] Whether the initiating figment is black or bright and blinding with the eyes open, it is subjectively blinding with the eyes closed, like a sheet of white paper in direct sunlight or phosphorous fireworks. Malakh elegizes, "[A] good catch-all for knowing what an aura is like would be to paint your telly screen with glitter nail polish and then watch *Yellow Submarine.*"[32] Sacks refers to it simply as an "elaborate hallucination within the visual field."[33]

Migraine auras are so transformational and fugitive that it is difficult to give an ordinary description of them. Many of the features I have described (or will describe) are seen by some migraineurs, while others perceive quite different patterns. My depiction is not a statistically average aura as much as a composite of many auras. People may experience these patterns in the same or different orders or may perceive another design altogether that nonetheless includes some of the elements I have listed or will list. Suffice it to say that everything I adduce is a component of a migraine aura, even if it does not occur in all auras or with the dynamics or sequence in which I present it.

Derek Robinson, migraine-aura curator, uses the description of a patient to characterize the elusiveness and variability of this phase,: "Like most other people suffering from migraine I get visual disturbances of course, and I've tried to depict these in my paintings, but it's a little difficult at times, as these patterns change in form; when you draw them you are really drawing only one form, or perhaps remembering them in a series that you put together.

"I've seen a flame … on several occasions; it's usually leaping about all the time—contracting and expanding like a living thing— like a sea anemone in fact.

"If the colors are strong, they're superimposed and tend to blot out my field of vision. On the other hand, the wavering grey patterns—they're like shimmers of light criss-crossing and swirling round each other—you can be right in the midst of these but still see through them. Then there are cellophane patterns. It's like watching shallow waves rippling across the sand. The ripple is there, yet you

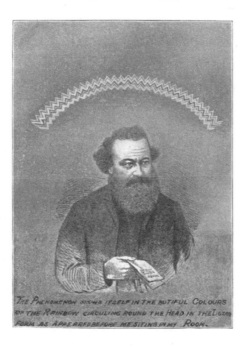

Figure 4: Somewhat fanciful placement of an arched spectrum with the colors of the rainbow (in the original) as represented by Mr. Beck. (From William Richard Gowers, *Subjective Sensations of Sight and Sound*, Philadelphia: P. K. Blakiston's Son & Co., 1904, p. 40.)

can see right through it and below it. These moving shadows and lights can be quite beautiful in fact. I'd love to see the northern lights, I've an idea they might be similar."[34]

Scotomata appear in both halves of the visual field, pulsing simultaneously, extending the overall disturbance to a half hour or so. There may also be "rippling, shimmering, and undulation" of a part or the whole of the visual field, "which patients may compare to wind-blown water, or looking through watered silk."[35] The landscape can also take on the appearance of a "waving, checked blanket."[36] "A particularly pleasing pattern," remarks Sacks, "is that of a spectrum in the form of an arch, centrally and bilaterally placed in the visual field. . . . Such a radiant [vault] was described by Aretaeus nearly two thousand years ago. . . ."[37]: "'flashes of purple or black colours before the sight, or all mixed together, so as to exhibit the appearance of a rainbow expanded in the heavens.'"[38] Others have described such an augment less pastorally as a canopy of luminous, vibrating, multicolored barbed wire.

As the scotoma erupts through the visual field, an opacity or eclipse follows its shimmering chevron, leaving a wake of sightlessness and/or image-bereft moils, probably the result of neurons being stunned by the overbrightness and hyperactivity of the excitation, hence shutting off. This so-called *negative scotoma,* perceived as loss of illumination and/or indistinct vision, like the scotoma occurs in *both* eyes simultaneously; thus is hemianopic.* Lashley deduces: "Whatever the precipitating cause of the disturbance, [the] facts indicate that an inhibitory process, in the case of the blind areas, or an excitatory process, in the case of the scintillations, is initiated in one part of the visual cortex and spreads over an additional area. As the process spreads, activity at the point where it was initiated is extinguished, and the process of extinction also spreads over the same area at about the same rate as does the active process."[39]

This zone may be "totally blind, amblyopic,† and/or outlined by scintillations."[40] When there is shadow, it is usually followed by a penumbra where sight is gradually being restored, like the faintly lit portion of a gibbous moon. The negative scotoma may be inseparable from the leading positive one or (rarely) precede it. Gowers elucidates:

"[T]he region of inhibition is also one of subdued discharge . . .

---

*Hemianopia (or hemiopia) is blindness in one half of the visual field of one or both eyes.

†Amblyopia is an enigmatic dimness of sight independent of change in the eye's structures, also known as lazy-eye blindness.

so that the area in which there is loss may present a dim luminosity, as if occupied by minute particles of luminous sand in constant molecular movement. In some cases the positive discharge is clearly primary and the inhibitory loss is secondary; in others the loss is primary and the luminous discharge is secondary. In the former the bright spectrum usually surrounds the area of dimness of sight; in the latter the primary (or simultaneous) dimness of sight extends to the edge of the field of vision and the discharge occurs within it.

"When seen in the dark, or with the eyes closed, the region nearest the limiting line, where the interference with sight is the greatest, presents a bright scintillation (see Figure 2, p. 13). . . . More careful scrutiny of this region of faint luminosity shows [as depicted in Figure 5, page 30] that in it there is a peculiar linear appearance; lines of luminosity are ranged parallel to the segments of the limiting spectrum, most distinct near to it. They have somewhat the semblance of internal reflections of the lines, becoming nearer and fainter as they recede from the limiting line, and they are more conspicuous in relation to some of the limiting lines than to others."[42] The bastioned structure of the margins of the negative scotoma or its interface with the normal visual image and/or positive aspect morphs in shape and color as it expands, a phase known as "buildup" and resembling "ramparts of a walled city . . . [giving] rise to the term *fortification spectra* (teichopsia)."[43] The spectral lines are refractory and usually nonconfluent, forming an acute angle, colored or gray, while continuing to oscillate in both position and brightness. Sacks mentions a "boiling movement or scintillation throughout the luminous portions of the scotoma. . . ."[44] Everything in them is moving, glimmering, unstable.

The characteristic shimmering or scintillation suggests an old-fashioned motion picture or flipbook which is slow enough that the individual frames no longer flow together seamlessly into scenery. "The rate of scintillation is below the flicker-fusion frequency, yet

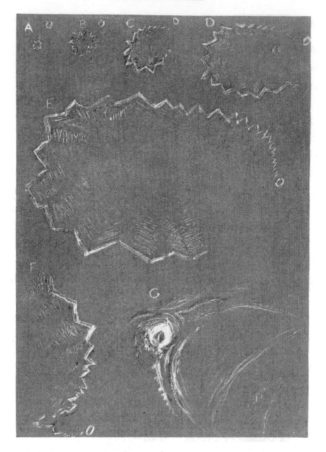

Figure 5: The chief elements of one of Airy's colored drawings (reduced), as expli-
cated by W. R. Gowers. "A bright stellate object, a small angled sphere, suddenly
appears in one side of the combined fields. In A it is seen a little to the left and
below the fixing-point O. It rapidly enlarges, first as a circular zigzag, but on the
inner side, toward the medial line, the regular outline becomes faint (B), and,
as the increase in size goes on, the outline here becomes broken (C), the gap
becoming larger as the whole increases, and the original circular outline becomes
oval. The form assumed is roughly concentric with the edge of the field of vision
so far as the lower and outer part of the oval is concerned, where the lines which
constitute the outline meet at right angles or larger angles. These remain large
and increase as the oval extends, their number and the number of angles continuing the same. The result bears some resemblance to the place of a fortification and hence it is sometimes called the 'fortification spectrum.' But (as seen
at E) the upper part of the zigzag oval presents a remarkable difference from the

too fast to count; its frequency has been estimated by indirect methods, as lying between 8 and 12 scintillations per second."[45]

Lashley analyzes the structure and expression of the striations: "The size of the fortification figures does not increase with increase in the size of the scotoma, but additional figures are added as the area grows.... The lines are of dazzling brightness, subjectively of the order of direct sunlight reflected from a white surface. They

rest. The position of the break is to leave the extremity of this close to the fixing-point of the field (O in all figures). The expansion above is at first less, so that the upper side is flatter, and the angles lessen progressively towards the fixing point. Near this they are scarcely to be discerned and at last are represented only by one or two luminous spots. When this angled oval has extended through the greater part of the half field (E) this upper portion also expands; it seems to overcome at last some resistance in the immediate neighborhood of the fixing-point, although close to it the stability seems too great to be overcome, so that a bulge occurs in the part above, and the angular elements of the outline here enlarge (as in F), although close to the fixing-point the line remains unchanged. After this final stage occurs, the outer lower part of the outline disappears."[41] (From William Richard Gowers, *Subjective Sensations of Sight and Sound*, Philadelphia: P. K. Blakiston's Son & Co., 1904, p. 24.)

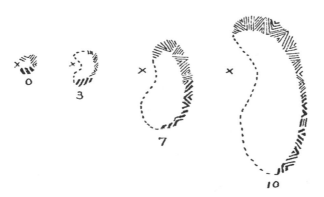

Figure 6: Sequential grids of a scintillating scotoma to show characteristic distribution of its fortification figures. The initial fixation point is marked each time by an X. (Karl Spencer Lashley, "Patterns of Cerebral Integration Indicated by Scotomas of Migraine," *Archives of Neurological Psychiatry*, 1941, Vol. 46, p. 334)

occur along the advancing margin of the area, followed by the blind region.... The scintillations have the form of distinct parallel lines, which cannot be counted but give the impression of groups of five or more. These seem to sweep across the figure toward the advancing margin and are constantly renewed at the inner margin, like the illusion of movement of a revolving screw...."[46]

Airy's account captures an unearthly scene: "When it was at its height it seemed like a fortified town with bastions all around it, these bastions being coloured most gorgeously.... All the interior of the fortification, so to speak, was boiling and rolling around in a most wonderful manner as if it was some thick liquid all alive."[47]

Gowers adds: "The lines which, in Dr. Airy's experience constituted the angled outline, varied in length, and the luminosity was broken or continuous at their junction; it was often bordered by a narrow dark line. Many of the angled lines presented conspicuous colours, bright red, dark blue, and yellow. The colour occupied the whole of one of the lines or only part of one. The same colour scarcely ever appeared on two adjacent lines. Red was followed usually by blue, sometimes by white, and often a white line had, as it were, a splash of colour in it. It is curious that green* was never seen, or at least it cannot have been conspicuous, since it was never remembered. The only general fact that can be discerned is that the contrast in direction is accompanied by a contrast in colour."[48]

Expanding in about three-quarters of the cases, the scotoma and the fortification spectra eventually drift toward the periphery of the visual field. Oscillating at ten pulses per second and dilating slowly, the morphology dances like a slow-moving blip on a radar screen[49] along the visual field at a pace of approximately 3 millimeters per

---

*Green was, however, reported by other migraineurs, as evident from other quotes in this book.

minute, as first measured by Lashley in the 1940s.[50] Progressing at this leisurely rate, it takes about twenty to thirty minutes (as noted subjectively by witnesses) to pass from its initiation point to the terminator of the visual field.

As it reaches the margin, the scintillation may boil or turn into spray, string, or a sensation of shooting stars as it dissipates entirely,[51] an activity noted above.

This is the full extent of many migraine auras, but some scotomata develop further and a few evolve into remarkably complex hallucinations.

Minor variations (identified below) are worth mentioning:

The period of aura excitation may include prickling, itching, and other forms of diffuse sensory arousal and excitation. The inhibition phase sometimes comprises not only blind spots (negative scotomata), but other sensory impoverishment: drowsiness, faintness, memory loss, and degrees of sensory deficit.

A scotoma may develop in a divergent part of the visual field from the original dot. A second scotoma may also emerge where the fixation point gave rise to the original one, even as it is fading. That is, a complete cycle may be followed by re-excitation and re-inhibition. Gowers describes a version of this: "A curious secondary spectrum was sometimes observed towards the end of the process. When the expanding angular outline had attained its maximum, a fresh stellate body was observed near the broken extremities, at or about the spot at which the first commenced and similar in aspect. Seen for a short time during the fading of the first spectrum, it then disappeared, having the semblance of an abortive attempt to repeat the process."[52]

A scotoma may also arise at a "normal" fixation point and, without developing or changing, circle the visual field, retracing its precise path once or twice and returning to the site of origin before "deciding" to angle off the edge of the visual field. Gowers also provides a variant of a radial scotoma*: "[A] stellate object ... unchanged throughout ... appeared usually near the edge of the right half of the field just below the horizontal line, and consisted of about six pointed leaflike projections, alternately red and blue (another example of contrasted colours in adjacent elements). It appeared on a small area of darkness [as shown in Figure 7, I]. This stellate body moved slowly towards the left and upwards, passing above the fixing-point, to a little beyond the middle line, then it returned to its starting place, retraced this path once or twice, and then passed to the right edge of the field at the lower outer part. Then it passed back again, only to a little beyond the spot at which it appeared, and then returned to the edge; after two or three repetitions of the last course it suddenly disappeared at the spot at which it commenced. The patient kept the eyes shut during its existence but on opening them when it had gone, always found that she could only see in the part of the field through which the spectrum had not passed. If she looked at a face a couple of feet from her she could only see the person's ear on the left side, and all that was to the right of the ear could not be seen; in only the third of the field to the left was there vision. The loss of sight lasted about a quarter of an hour, and gradually passed away."[53]

A third stage of migraine-aura organization, while varying dramatically by individual, is distinguished by highly complex, evolving geometric shapes, composite images, metamorphopsia (a visual hallucination that distorts the size, shape, and/or inclination of objects), meta-kaleidoscopic transformations of one configuration into another, and intimations of exotic scenery or the presence of mute visitors. The zigzags and bastions of the scintillating scotoma

---

*This particular aura will be discussed again later in the context of an epileptic replacement cycle.

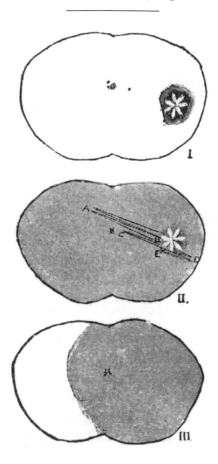

Figure 7: The mobile stellate scotoma of a patient who later developed epilepsy from a similar prodrome. (From William Richard Gowers, *Subjective Sensations of Sight and Sound,* Philadelphia: P. K. Blakiston's Son & Co., 1904, p. 32.)

may, for instance, next give rise to polygons which fuse or merge to form meshwork, spiderwebs, or lattices, which then spontaneously change scale, change color, change shape, change meaning. Triangles launch smaller triangles, and vortices break into scrolls which develop into fresh vortices as if a spiral object were spinning in place; these continue to compose themselves anew out of one another, becoming more complicated internally as they matriculate, rolling into their own margin as they are regenerated at their inner edge.*

Such effects evolve and mutate with a kind of manic and unforgiving intensity like a moving abstract-expressionist painting or a Walt Disney cartoon factory—Goofy or Bugs Bunny getting hit on the head repeatedly by a mallet. Sometimes before a shape can even be comprehended, another shape, bearing no relationship to it, has taken its place.

Sacks puts these phases in chronological and phenomenological context: "During or after the passage of simple phosphenes, some patients may observe, on closing the eyes, a form of visual tumult or delirium, in which latticed, faceted and tessellated motifs predominate.... These figments and elementary images tend to be brilliantly luminous, coloured, highly unstable, and prone to sudden kaleidoscopic transformations."[54]

Writer William Burrill declares, "Everything becomes surreal and yet so real. Like staring at a Cézanne or a Van Gogh. At four in the morning walking to the store you see art in the neighbor's garage. Your mind races and freeze-frames at the same time. Your eyes dazzle as if someone had popped a flashbulb in your face."[55]

A patient of Sacks notes, "[There were] patterns, as of Turkish carpets, suddenly changing. Images of flowers continuously raying and opening out. Everything faceted and multiplied: bubbles rising towards me, apertures opening and closing, honeycombs. These images are dazzling when I close my eyes, but still visible, more faintly, when the eyes are opened."[56]

In the most advanced stages of some migraine auras, there may be intricate moiré patterns and a generalized latticing of the field into more complex polygonal, often hexagonal sectors that granulate

---

*Once again, this description is a medley, comprising the third phases of many auras, and is unlikely to be the experience of any migraineur.

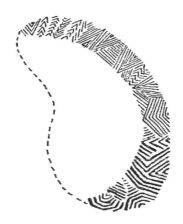

Figure 8: Sketch showing apparent modulation of texture and detail across a fortification. The thicker and more complicated designs are generally in the lower part of the field. (Karl Spencer Lashley, "Patterns of Cerebral Integration Indicated by Scotomas of Migraine," *Archives of Neurological Psychiatry,* 1941, Vol. 46, p. 335)

into smaller and yet smaller crystals. Fortifications may become finer and less intricate in their upper hemispheres but denser and more complicated at the bottom. If the spiderweb or latticing is thin, scenery and faces can be seen through it, giving a bizarre composite effect like tattoos on the world or landscapes being seen through a delicately embroidered veil. If the mosaic is thick, the rendition is like a cubist painting.

Sometimes the display morphs into distinct, very odd images: "small white skunks with erect tails, moving in procession across one quadrant of the visual field,"[57] or mice and rats.

The migraineur does not know whether there are real objects behind these hallucinations, as they may develop into entire landscapes with imaginary personages and events. One sufferer regularly encountered a figure clad in black seated with his back toward him or standing at a long table.[58] Another experienced his room suddenly filled with "red Indians" crowding around him. On a different occasion he picked up nonexistent musical instruments from the floor and began to play them.[59]

These mirages and phantasmagoria are referred to by Sacks as "synthetic or imaginary geographies…, pseudogeographies … created by the excited brain."[60]

Deformations of visual/kinesthetic reality and metamorphopsias may encompass: dimensionless flattening of objects as if into two-dimensional pancakes without tactile depth; distortion of object contours; exaggeratedly sharp contours or brilliant, fiery outlines; monocular and binocular diplopias (double vision); bright and inappropriate colors, color changes, or complete loss of color; loss of contrast discrimination; "waviness of linear components in visual images and formation of concentric halos …, eccentric misplacements in the visual field";[61] and distortions of size in relation to perspective or total loss of scale. Less typical variations include multiple vision, the apparent movement of stationary objects, and the division of the visual field into two disaffiliated parts. Muleksis tells his chatroom: "My aura … divides my sight into two, horizontally. And the lower bit (it is not half-half when it starts, the lower part is smaller) gives me a 'shaking image.' As if you are looking over the flames and see a transparent layer between you and the world that 'shakes.'"[62] In inverted vision (sometimes called reversal-of-vision metamorphopsia), a rare symptom, the visual field rotates 180 degrees in the coronal plane.

Advanced auras can also elicit zoom vision whereby objects spontaneously enlarge and diminish, draw close and then shoot far away. Dysmetria, an inability to gauge distance correctly, also accompanies some auras.

In their complex transfigurations, auras leap across sense boundaries and often comprise "intense affective states, deficits and disturbances of speech and ideation, dislocations of space- and time-perception, and a variety of dreamy, delirious, and trancelike states."[63] These disorientations and deficiencies, sometimes approaching delirium, resemble other kinds of trances, fugues, and transient amnesias.

Quasi-visual and extra-visual effects are myriad: broken and stuttering speech, confusion regarding visually guided hand movements, false gauging of distance, difficulty in remembering familiar words, perception or identification of the wrong object, starting one story and finishing with another, and isolation of objects in the visual field so that they stand out one by one but do not become part of the field as a whole (see below). The left and right sides of reality, including objects held in each hand, make no sense in relation to each other. Ordinary objects appear unfamiliar (visual agnosia). An object hidden or distorted behind a blind spot may be relocated when the head is turned, but it *may be perceived* as not having been there in the first place.

Lashley analyzes the odd discontinuity of blind spots and intermittent fields: "A negative scotoma may completely escape observation, even when it is just off the macula, unless it obscures some object to which attention is directed. Talking with a friend, I glanced just to the right of his face, whereon his head disappeared. His shoulders and necktie were still visible, but the vertical stripes in the wallpaper behind him seemed to extend right down to the necktie. Quick mapping revealed an area of total blindness covering about 30 degrees, just off the macula. It was quite impossible to see this as a blank area when projected on the striped wall or other uniformly patterned surface, although any intervening object failed to be seen."[64]

Words lose their ordinary meanings or cannot be found in the mind (anomia). Or a blatantly incorrect name is used, such as calling a pot a spoon (semantic paraphasia). One patient notes: "I'd find myself using the wrong words—completely nonsensical words ... and my speech was slurred, as if I was drunk...."[65]

Some migraineurs see expressionless faces or faces that are not faces; meanwhile they do not recognize familiar people because their countenances do not look familiar; even their names no longer seem legitimate. No wonder Oliver Sacks' renowned subject "mistook his wife for a hat." Though probably not undergoing a prolonged aura (no final diagnosis was ever made), this patient suffered from the chronic inability to recognize certain objects as what they were (or even as commonplace), a disorder known as prosopagnosia. His misperceptions indicate how defects in the visual cortex (their likely source) can give rise to cognitive distortions and wide-ranging lapses of meaning. Referred to Sacks in an ophthalmic context, this gentleman actually grasped his wife's head at the end of the session and then attempted to put it on his own. During the preceding interview he seemed to assemble the world by moving his attention from feature to feature rather than grasping it as a whole. At another meeting he did not recognize the rose in Sacks' lapel as a flower, instead seeing it as a "red convoluted pattern."[66]

Advanced migrainous sensations also have a timeless quality, as if they will never end: "an extraordinary sense of stillness came upon me, a feeling that I had lived this moment before, in the same place.... I felt that this summer afternoon had always existed, and that I was arrested in an endless moment."[67] There may be extreme *déjà vu* (haunting familiarity) and *jamais vu* (inexplicable strangeness or unfamiliarity). During an aura, a past event may come back so vividly as to fuse with the present world and displace consciousness. There is sometimes an intimation of being more than one person or having access to separate minds. In that sense auras are not only *dys*functions but uncoordinated fragments of paranormal functions (see pp. 138–139).

In other instances it seems as though time stops during the scotoma's passage or, even stranger, that time keeps stopping and starting over again. Time may also seem to be progressing in slow motion or at sonic speed. Some have felt as though they were acting with absurd haste or, contrarily, at a snail's pace while others were jabbering away too hurriedly to be understood.

Sensations of strangeness and disorganization may involve dyslexia and dysphasia and result in doing things backwards, getting things out of order, and/or exaggerated clumsiness, slurred speech, and spastic responses.

Unable to do anything else useful during an aura, one author tried to write a simple family letter longhand, only to discover afterward that he had composed completely different words and thoughts than he remembered.[68] It was as though a different member of a "multiple personality" had taken over without his being aware of it.

A few people experience magnification or diminution of their own body image. A region of anatomy may feel enlarged, shrunken, misshapen (dysmorphic) or absent altogether. One migraineur reported feeling very small, "about a foot high," whereas another suddenly sensed that the right half of his body had become twice as dense or large as the left. Yet another sufferer protested that her left ear was "ballooning out six inches or more."[69] The patient reported by Robinson marveled: "[T]here were times when I thought that my hands and arms were so enormous that they touched the floor and I had to keep looking at them to convince myself they were the right size. I couldn't help wondering then if anyone else would notice—but I don't suppose they ever did." Meanwhile, "sounds seemed to impinge on my skin and I'd try to brush them off with my enormous hands."[70] Such impaired epidermal sensations are known as paresthesias.

One woman confided an unusual dystopia to her doctor: "I experienced the sensation that my head had grown to tremendous proportions and was so light that it floated up to the ceiling, although

I was sure it was still attached to my neck. I used to try to hold it down with my hands. This sensation would pass with the migraine but would leave me with a feeling that I was very tall."[71] She couldn't forbear looking in the mirror to make sure this wasn't objectively true even though rationally she knew it was a hallucination.

Phenomena in the external world may become surreally large or surreally small, sometimes in succession. A migraineur whose aura imposed itself onto a book he was reading experienced the page as "like the furrows in a ploughed field.... I could see them between the lines of the book ... but the book looked huge, and the furrows seemed like great chasms, hundreds of feet behind the lines of print."[72]

Sacks refers to these changes elegantly as Brobdignagian and Lilliputian, respectively.[73] In a Lilliputian hallucination, the scenery is reduced to the scale of a miniature crystal ball, the sort of souvenir world that is shaken to create the appearance of a snowfall; this can be breathtakingly beautiful, as novelist Siri Hustvedt recounts in a migraine with Lilliputian characters:

"I was lying in bed one afternoon, very happily reading Italo Svevo. For some reason, I looked down at the floor beside me and there were two small pink figures—a man and an ox. I would say they were between six and seven inches tall and despite their odd color, highly articulated and life-like. They walked and gestured. I distinctly remember the man reaching down to pet the ox, but neither of them acknowledged me. Oddly, the apparition didn't alarm me in the least, and I don't remember thinking that I was having an aura. The two fascinated and pleased me, and I wanted to keep looking and looking at the enchanted creatures that had arrived on the floor of my bedroom. It's hard to estimate, but I would think that the hallucination lasted for perhaps two minutes. The vision was followed by a headache, but not a terribly severe one."[74]

Disorientations of memory, time, and space; auditory, olfactory, and gustatory hallucinations; various dystopias and paresthesias all express Boolean equivalence to the scotoma and confirm that its visual and cephalgic aspects are the tip of an iceberg. In essence, while a scintillating motif is propagated across the ocular cortex, a spasm is discharging across other tissues. The more diverse cortical area it captures, apparently the greater the range of neurological, neuropsychological, and parapsychological artifacts it generates.

Historical and Artistic Legacy of Migraines

Ancient and Medieval References

No doubt from the Stone Ages among hominids—in fact likely among all animals with brains—migraine auras have occurred and been regarded as existential events; i.e., as real in the environment or spirit world.

Other than possibly some aura-like rock art and geometric ornaments in cave paintings, records of migraines begin with a set of Babylonian tablets from 2000–1880 B.C. which contain priests' dialogues with the gods in Neo-Sumerian concerning incantations against migraine.[75] Auras were so-named by Pelops, teacher of the famous second-century A.D. Roman physician Galen, who called them pneumatic vapors *(pneumatika aura)* in keeping with Greek elemental theory[76] whereby a mixture of humors gives rise to a living organism in which they then vary over a lifetime in states of balance and imbalance, health and disease. Pelops' astute discernment of the humoral characteristics of migraine auras has been overlooked or relegated to secondary status in recent times—the phenomenon does in fact resemble a damp spirit (an airy vapor) rising spasmodically through the viscera to the head.

Although there is a very spotty history of migraines subsequently through the centuries, at least the notorious headaches have been mentioned by Hippocrates, Julius Caesar, Aretaeus, the apostle Paul, Miguel de Cervantes, and England's Queen Mary, as well as many others. In instances where a dissociated visual hallucination has been recorded we are unable to tell whether it originated in migraine or some other psychophysiological or hallucinogenic source. In fact, our most substantial records of possible auras from early historical times come from their conflation with religious visions, as they share aspects with spirit encounters, states of possession, messages from God and, later, UFOs and alien abductions (see pp. 121–122). Did Joan of Arc experience auras or autonomous visions?

Although the phenomena hailed by twelfth-century nun Hildegard of Bingen have been classified as religious epiphanies and were described by her as coming from God, they almost certainly were migraine auras:

"I saw a great star most splendid and beautiful, and with its exceeding multitude of falling stars which with the star followed southwards.... And suddenly they were all annihilated, being turned into black coals ... and cast into the abyss so that I could see them no more....

"The light which I see is not located, but yet is more brilliant than the sun, nor can I examine its height, length or breadth, and I name it 'the cloud of the living light.' ...

"Sometimes I behold within this light another light which I name 'the Living Light itself.'"[77]

But then who is to say that a migraine aura cannot also be an autonomous intelligence or an angelic light?

Eighteenth- through Twentieth-Century Mentions

It is believed that Emily Dickinson was partly describing a classic migraine when she wrote: "The nail's in the coffin,/And full fathom five we lie,/With rings on our fingers,/And diamonds in our eyes." The poem continues in a conjecturally migrainous vein, "Redeem the dream that is now hidden.... /Do not these sirens believe."[78]

The account by Lewis Carroll (aka Charles L. Dodgson) of the land Alice entered by following a rabbit down a hole is thought by some to have been inspired by his auras. One paper cites "inexplicable similarities between the experiences described in the two Alice books and the semeiology of migraine aura symptoms both in the visual and somesthetic domain."[79] Certain events in Alice's travels seem so provocatively migrainous that, three years after the resemblance was documented by C. W. Lippman in the *Journal of Nervous and Mental Disease* (1952), a roster of these adventures was consigned collectively to "Alice in Wonderland Syndrome" or AWS by John Todd in the *Canadian Medical Association Journal*. In addition to the core feature of body image disturbances, AWS includes the false orientation of objects in space, the multiplication of one entity into two or more, impaired sense of time, visual inversion,[80] visual-field rotation, geographical detachment, disorientations of kinesthesia, aphasia, language disturbances, and metamorphoses of personages into humanoid creatures or talking animals.[81] Though likely an overdeterminism of parallel elements married to a lack of metaphorical imagination, AWS hyperbole is worth indulging for a few paragraphs.

The most scotoma-like aspect of *Alice in Wonderland* is the palinopsian Cheshire-Cat of whom Alice remarked, "Well! I've often seen a cat without a grin. But a grin without a cat! It's the most curious thing I've ever seen in my life."

Kinesthetic influences of hallucinogens as well as migraines are epitomized by the Caterpillar who, after finishing its smoke and taking its hookah out of its mouth, wanders away, telling Alice as it yawns: "One side will make you grow smaller, and the other side will make you grow larger."

Even as Alice is wondering, "One side of what?" the Caterpillar says, as if she had asked the question aloud, "'Of the mushroom....'

In another moment it was out of sight."[82]

AWS is exemplified by other exotic features: cryptozooids like the Mock Turtle and Gryphon, feeling short and wide like Tweedle-Dum and Tweedle-Dee, being blinded by a light as Alice is by the Moon, the sensation of a fall (down a rabbit hole) that does not seem to end, Humpty-Dumpty's poor arithmetic in *Through the Looking Glass* (acalculia), the uncertainty of whether one is awake or dreaming, hallucination of voices (the Rabbit and mice ordering Alice around), Alice's sonic flight with the Red Queen, anomia (surprise at not being able to think of a word) while talking to the Fawn, phoneme substitutions ("pig for fig"), and unpleasantly repetitive *déjà vu* (an old song ringing through her head like the ticking of a clock). Other auditory distortions include sounds coming from weird places like under a tree, sounds converting back and forth between noise and words (the snoring of the Queens), the Lion's voice like a bell, the Beetle's distorted hoarse/horse voice, silent and distant voices, disembodied choruses of voices, the cooing of the White Queen like a pigeon in *Through the Looking Glass,* and her later speech which became so loud, shrill, and whistlelike that Alice had to hold her hands over her ears.[83]

The entire chess game in *Through the Looking Glass* is rife with elements of absent-mindedness (the character-pieces) and defective philosophico-logical rationalizations indicative of migraine.[84]

Sometime in the late 1850s Dodgson drew an elfin figure in his notebook, a lad skillfully rendered except that part of his face, shoulders, wrist, and hand are missing, covered on their right with a "rounded border" defect exactly like that of a negative scotoma. Elsewhere, he wrote that he had "experienced, for the second time, that odd optical affection of seeing moving fortifications followed by a headache,"[85] a classical migraine. Yet nowhere does he openly identify the sketch or his novels with the condition.

My opinion is that Carroll/Dodgson is unconsciously representing not so much migraine auras as the much larger and less pre-scriptive migrainoid* world that had not been delineated in his time—in fact, most of the educated populace is still unaware of it. While *Alice in Wonderland* and *Through the Looking Glass* more or less invoke migrainoid situations, almost assuredly they were not written to depict them. After all, it does not take an active migraine condition or experience of auras for people to to visit the nonsense realms of hallucinatory and symbolic logic.

Where art, neuropathology, religious visions, fairy tales, sur-realism, and freelance word-play and semeiology overlap, aspects of many realms can be represented simultaneously without an alle-giance to one over the others. This seems a more reasonable expla-nation for Dodgson's narrative landscape than that a nonmedical man chose to write a pair of elaborate parables as his private migraine cryptic.

If we are to believe some of the popular post-modern accounts of Dodgson's fantasies such as the 1986 movie *Dreamchild,* then we might attribute the fantastic elements of AWS to the sublimation and displacement of Dodgson's love for the real-life child Alice, a passion so unthinkable and tabooed as to express itself only in the most grotesquely melancholy and deviant landscapes and charac-ters. In such a representational realm a fairy tale of migrainoid fan-tasies becomes a cover or rebus-like code for repressed pedophilia and unrequited love. AWS is better explained as an illicit seduction and semi-erotic (but virginal) "molestation" of a child with whom an adult was infatuated.

The putative first depiction of medical images of migraine auras appeared in 1845 in the form of various scintillating scotomata in a German ophthalmological textbook by Christian Georg Theodor

---

*See pp. 114–116 for a definition and explanation of this term.

Ruete. Several decades later Jean Marie Charcot (1888), Joseph Jules Franáois Félix Babinski (1890), and Sir William Richard Gowers (1895) drew variants of phosphenes, dancing rows of triangles, fortification spectra, arched rainbows, and other migrainous artifacts see Figures 1, 2, 4, and 5).

The Dutch impressionist Vincent Van Gogh may have suffered from migraines (one presumes these were classical ones with auras), although this claim has not been substantiated by scholarly analyses of his life and work from a pathographic point of view. He painted "Starry Night" with its whorling celestial objects surrounded by halations while being treated for "Migraine Personality" at the St. Remy Asylum in France in 1889. His sunflowers and irises also have a "migrainoid" ring to them.[86]

It is believed (with a similar lack of substantiating studies) that the French impressionist Georges Seurat experienced visual auras too and that the pointillistic technique he employed in most of his oils, for instance "Courbevoie Bridge" (1886), was conveyed to him, at least in part, by his migraines. Other vaguely scotoma-suggestive images include gliding and idle boats, smoking factory-chimneys, carnival actors, bathers, groves of trees, river banks, mirror-like water, laterally oriented figures, strollers with umbrellas, stylized shadows and, in general, broad, smooth layered strokes and vibrant, slightly inaccurate colors and contrasts. The torpid, still mood of many of these canvasses suggests the timelessness of an aura. In some neurological writing, the scintillating scotoma is immortalized as the "Seurat Effect," which may be another case of overzealous literalism.[87]

Pablo Picasso denied ever having migraine auras; yet his cubist-period work beginning in the late 1930s has a look so migrainous that the terms "cubist" and "Picasso-like" have become more official designations for migraine than "the Seurat Effect." "The Weeping Woman," "The Portrait of Woman with Hat," and "Guernica" are all quasi-migrainous blueprints with their fracturing and mosaic repatterning of faces along vertical axes such that one eye is higher than its counterpart and adjoining features are distorted and disproportioned as in a cartoon. In fact, the central image on the cover of Oliver Sacks' *Migraine*—a man's face and clothing turning into mosaics reminiscent of a pig- or dog-headed humanoid—is an overt tribute to "The Weeping Woman."* Picasso himself attributed his cachet variously to "painting forms as he thought rather than saw them," the violence of the Spanish Civil War, and African tribal art.[88] But who is to say that traditional African figurines did not gestate their migrainous traits through a long, prehistoric lineage?

The discussion becomes tautological. It is not possible or even important to resolve whether any particular images are migraine-influenced, as a migrainoid aesthetic radiates through a far wider variety of sources and forms than just clinical migraines. "Migraine" is a way of viewing the universe, which may be imposed by a bioneural sequence but can also occur through other, quite disparate channels. The outlook has its own style and signature extrinsic of its biology. Among other graphic artists whose work is related, either explicitly or inherently, to migraines are Giorgio de Chirico, Salvador Dali, Yayoi Kusama, Marina Abramovic, and Sarah Raphael.

In the late twentieth and early twenty-first centuries migraine art has developed as its own genre from the rationale that migraines can be more accurately depicted by images than words. This portfolio constitutes not a mode of neurological imaging or "migraine handwriting" but illustrations of diverse media and styles representing, by either realism or abstraction, the experience of headaches and auras. The growing body of work enables indescribable symptoms to be shared among migraineurs, while non-migraineurs

---

*From the collection of the Migraine Action Association (see below).

can intuit what sufferers undergo beyond myths and hearsay. Samples of this art can be found in galleries, exhibitions, publications, and on websites (www.migraine-org/EN/Migraine.Art.html).

The originator of the Migraine Art concept, Derek Robinson, was a career marketing executive with Boehringer Ingelheim Limited, a multinational pharmaceutical company, when he unwittingly started a second career in 1973 by soliciting graphic material for his company's advertising campaign promoting a new drug for migraine prevention. Eventually he was led to a British Midlands teacher who illustrated her own auras for her family doctor. Robinson borrowed some of those images for the campaign. Six years later, with the marketing long concluded, he was contacted by Peter Wilson, founder of the British Migraine Association, to help publicize its mission in a similar manner.[89]

Believing that there might be others who sketched or painted their migraines, Robinson helped to launch four National Migraine Art competitions (1980–1987)—a curation technique later imitated in the United States. The first competition, jointly sponsored by the British Migraine Association and WB Pharmaceuticals Limited, proposed three submission categories: visual auras, pain, and the effect of migraines on an artist's life. Approximately 900 entries came from all over the world, including several from children. After the judgings, selected exhibitions toured England. The Migraine Art collection was maintained by Robinson until his death in 2001 and is now archived by the Migraine Action Association; as of late June 2004, it comprises 562 works not returned by request to their artists.[90]

American exhibitions of similar vignettes include "The Art of Migraine," sponsored by the Faulkner Hospital in Boston in 1987, and "Mosaic Vision," a selection of 90 creative works of migraine at the Exploratorium in San Francisco in 1991. A visitor to the latter wrote: "[W]hen I saw a visual record of what other migraineurs

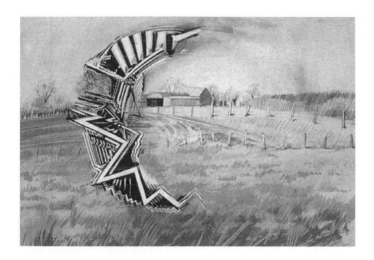

Figure 9: Artist's rendering of a scotoma with fortifications over a farm (original in color). Migraine Art is reproduced by permission of the Migraine Action Association and Boheringer Ingelheim UK Limited.

went through, I had an incredible relief, that I wasn't the only one. Many of the images were so disturbing that I felt grateful that my migraines aren't that intense."[91] She added that she took her husband, a non-sufferer, to the show, and it was the first time he had an appreciation of her lot. Another woman wrote: "[I]t was just what I had been trying to describe! We are in this together."[92]

Subsequent Migraine Art shows have been curated in Oberhausen, Germany (1997), and Skien, Norway (2004).

Dr. Klaus Podoll, a migraine researcher at the University Clinic of Aachen in Germany and Robinson's aesthetic heir, has co-authored two books on migraine art: *Migraine and Spiritual Experience* with Robinson himself and *The Aura of Giorgio de Chirico: Migraine Art and Metaphysical Art* with Ubaldo Nicola. He is the current overseer for submissions of art to a *Migraine Art in the Internet* module maintained on the Migraine Aura Foundation's website.[93]

Musicians suffering from migraine run a gamut from Gustav Mahler and Peter Tchaikovsky to Elvis Presley and Loretta Lynn, and include Charles Gounod, Edith Frost, Carly Simon, and Jeff Tweedy of the alternative country band Wilco, who referred to songs that "start out quietly and end in complete disorder—a form of musical entropy."[94]

The following catalogue is of pop-migrainous interest courtesy of the Migraine Aura Foundation:

• Marilyn Manson's equivalent to a liner note: "A postcard from the migraine fields. So we will now return our efforts to the melolagnia at hand. DRUMS!!! (Doctor's orders.) From the migraine fields, MM"[95];

• the CD "Chance Meeting of a Defective Tape Machine and Migraine," Nurse With Wound, 2003[96];

• the words, *"No pain no gain migraine ..."* from the CD "Abrasive" by the group Puddle of Mudd, 2001[97];

• the song "Migraine" from the CD "Broken Airplanes" by Troubled Hubble (2001) with the lines: *"I saw my mom floored, on her knees/begging lord oh lord/take away this pain from me/I saw my mom floored, on her knees begging lord oh lord/can you help me please."*[98]

Members of the hall-of-fame of "outed" migraineurs include Napoleon Bonaparte, Thomas Jefferson, Immanuel Kant, Friedrich Nietzsche, Edgar Allen Poe, possibly William Blake, Robert E. Lee, Ulysses S. Grant (in fact he experienced one on the day he accepted Lee's surrender—no record as to whether Lee did too but, as we shall see, the victor is more likely to suffer a migraine than the vanquished), also Sigmund Freud, Karl Marx, Alexander Graham Bell, Virginia Wolfe, Georgia O'Keeffe, Marvin Minsky, and John F. Kennedy. Among contemporary performers and athletes are Elizabeth Taylor, Whoopi Goldberg, Elle Macpherson, Dwight Gooden, Fred Couples, José Canseco, and Terrell Davis (who had to sit out part of a Super Bowl because of a migraine). It is unknown how many of these had auras as well as headaches but, with a little imagination, one can locate scotomata and dysphasia in Kant's ontologies, Poe's nightmare landscapes and malign characters, O'Keeffe's abstractions and huge detailed, colorful flowers, and Elvis' "scintillating" stage performances. O'Keeffe, for one, explained some of her paintings as renderings of migraines: "It was a very bad headache ... why not do something with it?"[99]

At greater length the essayist Joan Didion portrayed the effects of her own classical migraines: "Once an attack is under way ... no drug touches it. Migraine gives some people mild hallucinations, temporarily blinds others, shows up not only as a headache but as a gastrointestinal disturbance, a painful sensitivity to all sensory stimuli, an abrupt overpowering fatigue, a strokelike aphasia, and a crippling inability to make even the most routine connections. When I am in a migraine aura (for some people the aura lasts fifteen minutes, for others several hours), I will drive through red lights, lose the house keys, spill whatever I am holding, lose the ability to focus my eyes or frame coherent sentences, and generally give the appearance of being on drugs, or drunk. The actual headache, when it comes, brings with it chills, sweating, nausea, a debility that seems to stretch the very limits of endurance. That no one dies of migraine seems, to someone deep into an attack, an ambiguous blessing."[100]

A Phenomenon that Gets Little Attention

Despite their commonness and frequency, migraine auras have become an enigma. A majority of people in the West have either never heard of them or, if they have, do not know their nature, degree of seriousness, or ubiquity. Most people who have experienced their spontaneous distortions of vision have no name for these and have gotten no diagnosis. Even most medical doctors understand them only as some sort of transient neurological artifact.

A scientist friend of mine who has done forty years of the highest-level research into the nervous system and its disorders declined an invitation to help with this volume, emailing me: "I have absolutely nothing to say about migraine auras except to describe my own, which are totally boring."

This conveys the current view that, whatever migraine auras are, they are biologically trivial.

Given that, at very least, a meaningful minority of the population experiences migrainous hallucinations and also that these artifacts render sufferers unable to function to one degree or another, they are understudied and underdiscussed. They have been paid even less attention in the last fifty years than in the preceding century and are now pretty much absent from not only most medical dialogue but also, astonishingly, gossip and small talk, which tend to encompass everything, whether earth-shattering or trivial.

How many people actually experience auras? Migraine statistics, especially those specifying auras, are subjective and speculative because most episodes go unreported and there are no measurable diagnostic protocols for them anyway. Basically the same queries about the same phenomena, depending on the method of interviewing, the era in which the data were collected, and the means of quantifying oral testimony, classify migraineurs as ranging from a small minority to almost everyone at one time or another.[101]

Current (2006) medical statistics for the United States offer roughly these demographics: 28 million Americans suffer chronic migraines; 12 percent experience migraines (with or without auras) in any one year; 10 percent get *auras* at least on occasion over their lifetimes; 10 percent suffer from migraine headaches without auras; 2 percent experience classical migraines. Women migraineurs (irrespective of auras) outnumber men by three to one, and the ratio is four to one during childbearing years (suggesting a hormonal co-factor); the majority of women also seems to be increasing; 25 percent of auras occur in people between the ages of thirty and forty, making this the peak group. Migraines are generally thought of as a post-puberty event, with the incidence in children at about 4 percent (though these are the least reliable specifiers, given the phantasmagoria already in their imaginations).[102]

Sacks cites a study by W. C. Alvarez published (1960) in *The American Journal of Ophthalmology* in which 12 percent of 618 male interviewees reported an experience of "a solitary scotoma."[103] Alvarez also interviewed 44 physicians, a sophisticated group, of whom an astonishing 87 percent reported experiencing "many solitary scotomata with never a headache."[104] Some Internet surveys since 2000 have corroborated this finding: 90 percent of randomly selected interviewees, once an aura was depicted to them, had memory of at least one occurrence with or without a headache. Many people had their sole headacheless aura in the distant past, perhaps during childhood, did not know what it was and forgot about it.

In my own seeking of accounts for this book, I found that more than half the people to whom I talked who initially said that they never had a visual aura reconsidered later. My attention jogged their memory. Typically they recollected a Sunday maybe fifteen years ago, maybe thirty-five years ago, when, while turning around in the bedroom or during a picnic in the park, they experienced a flash that wouldn't go away, followed by a distortion of objects and partial blindness. One fifty-year-old man suddenly recalled a solitary aura at the dinner table when he was twelve. It never happened again, and gradually he stopped thinking about it.

Another person, who had heard about scotomata for years, wished he had had one so that he could know what they were like. Then out of blue he remarked, "Could those bright shapes that crossed my vision in kindergarten have been migraine auras? They left me blinded for a while. I assumed that they were another of those things I wasn't supposed to understand. My teachers were no help on anything else, so I never told them. By George, I guess I had them! I remember the last one was at school around first or second grade. I was amazed no one else talked about this stuff; I figured maybe it was only me. I haven't had one for sixty years."

It is striking that, despite knowing full well that an aura consists of flashing shapes and blind spots, this man didn't identify his own singular experience of *precisely that symptom*. This is likely because the subjective experience of a scotoma is so obscure, transient, and personal that it relates to nothing in consensus reality, not even to a description of its own particulars. Though a dazzling pageant in full regalia, it is also a dysphasic mirage without sequel or meaning. Eventually most people forget that it happened to them and that it wasn't their imagination or a dream. There is neither context for its continued retention nor physical consequence to reinforce it.

Sacks cites a conversation with a zoologist colleague who responded to a diagram of a scintillating scotoma with instant recognition: "I often had it as a young man, usually when I was in bed at night. I was delighted by the colours and their expansion—it reminded me of the opening of a flower. It was never succeeded by a headache or other symptoms. I presumed everybody saw such things—it never occurred to me that it was a 'symptom' of anything."[105]

Auras are almost always isolated crises, well along the way to being over by the time the flashing shapes and blind spots are at their peak—terse, superficial breakdowns in normal bodily functioning, like persistent after-images or a variety of aches, cramps, and nonlocal pains and spells of dizziness that may momentarily be of concern but come and go quickly and do not return. Scotomata are also, as I shall soon discuss, marginally to acutely traumatizing, and trauma tends to blot out memory.

This apparent contradiction—too trivial to remember, yet too frightening to remember—explains a lot about auras: Something that is traumatic and major, like sexual violation or mutilation in war, is invariably remembered, especially by an older child or adult; it is too vivid to forget. Something that is traumatic and incidental has not only a pretext to become unconscious (its triviality) but a numbing barrier (its trauma). Whereas other minor events come and go in the memory neutrally (and thus can sometimes be summoned from the depths of oblivion if prompted), auras may be sealed out by their eeriness and disturbing charge. Declared by the psyche not to have happened or not to be important, they become a nonevent.

My wife experienced a scotoma while pouring tea in the kitchen during July 2002 at age fifty-eight, none before and none since, and the experience is now so indistinct in her mind that she has almost completely forgotten what she saw or what it felt like; she cannot relate to my own auras. She would not remember the occurrence at all if not for my involvement in the topic.

My conclusion is: a majority of people have isolated migraine auras and forget them, making the actual percentage of the population who experience them at one time or another unquantifiably high.

A full discussion of why migraine auras are unrecognized, misidentified, and misunderstood would require an investigation into social mores, cultural taboos, neurolinguistics, and semantics.

A first reason is, as noted, their lack of context and cogency; they do not have a place in standard mnemonic figuration.

Dreams suffer a similar fate nowadays, especially by comparison to the interest in them among other cultures and during earlier centuries in European culture. Yet dreams engender a wealth of literature and discussion by comparison with auras. Of course, dreams have generative, imaginative content and roots in more accessible psychospiritual landscapes than auras—yet auras belong to their class of relatively undervalued neuro-iconographies.

A second reason is their brevity and medical insignificance. A malaise lasting only about thirty minutes, with no apparent consequences of import and lacking a traceable connection to other illness, has no status in either modern neurological research or in people's daily considerations of their health. A doctor tells a patient that he or she has a visual migraine, the patient wonders what to do about it, and the doctor answers: "Nothing." Migraine auras are random, paroxysmal events—clinical without being pathological.

When a physical condition is not an omen of debilitating or fatal disease, does not impede or improve one's love life, does not cause chronic depression or panic attacks, and does not deter career advancement or accumulation of wealth, it is put on the back burner or left off the stove entirely.

Thirdly, misdiagnosis (or nondiagnosis) contributes to migraine auras' outcast status. There is currently no x-ray indicator or blood test for migraine (with or without auras). Diagnosis must be qualitative, historical, and epistemological, based on interpreting a patient's narrative. Further investigation (imaging by MRI or CT scan) is uncalled for unless headaches and/or scotomata are unusually severe and prolonged or occur suddenly in a person with suspicion of other neurological pathology. Even then it is difficult to know where to look and what to look for.

For instance, let's say a first-time sufferer undergoes an impromptu distortion of sight; he or she presumes an eye problem and makes an appointment with an ophthalmologist. Whereas many with migraine headaches call on a neurologist or general practitioner first, auras (MAWOHs) are reported most frequently in ophthalmic practices.

Multiple circumstances may preclude an eye-doctor's accurate diagnosis. First of all, migraine auras are so brief that the disturbance has vanished long before the patient arrives in the examination room, maybe even before he makes a phone call for an appointment.

Secondly, though ophthalmologists are familiar enough with auras to identify their symptoms instantly, some may, out of long-reinforced habit to first rule out serious pathologies, search fruitlessly with their instruments in the eyes for an agency. Their imprimatur is to make sure the person has nothing sight-threatening going on. The doctor then might tell the patient, as my original guy did, that they can find no *ophthalmic* condition. As far as neurological complications go, they may not want to make a guess, for reasons of professional integrity or from fear of liability. Even a neurological referral may be disappointing in getting an explanation or treatment for the condition. In the halfbakery chatroom Muleksis remarks curtly: "Ophthalmologist said nothing wrong with the eyes; neurologist said, if it happens about once a week we should suppress it with medication, but she could not explain what harm it would do if we didn't."[106]

In addition, unless the description of the aura is highly detailed and meticulously accurate, any doctor may ignore it as incidental or be misled to search for other causes: abnormalities in the cornea, lens, vitreous body, and retina; pathologies of the brain or vascular system; or external agents, all of which can incite aura-like symptoms. Incidental and environmental causes include reflections from corrective lenses, room lighting, car headlights, or stray light viewed peripherally. We will explore many of these pathologies and contingencies later (see pp. 151–153).

Eight years before I did my web search, I saw a different, quite sophisticated ophthalmologist for a case of shingles affecting my vision and, when he asked about my general eyesight, I described my auras. I got a baffled response; he cocked his head as though scanning his internal reference library and then frowned, "I don't know what that is." When I asked him if it could be a form of migraine, he concurred, nodding with affable sincerity: "It might well be." Yet it bore no further inquiry. Since I did not have that problem while he was treating a more acute one, neither of us mentioned it again.

In sum, ophthalmologists tend to be narrow-banded onto more dramatic retinal maladies and other ocular diseases like glaucoma, macular degeneration, and cataracts or, in league with optometrists, are intent on prescribing glasses to improve vision, so they give short shrift to migrainous symptoms.

In fact, I have been told of a few instances of scotomata being initially conflated ophthalmologically with vitreous "floaters" (bits of loose debris in the vitreous fluid of the cornea that clutter the field of vision of most people, to a greater or lesser degree, as they get older). The diagnosis of floaters is so common and even popular nowadays in the United States with an aging population that auras, though sharing few of the debris' cellular characteristics, get lost in their catchall category. Since most floaters are considered about as significant medically as warts or dandruff, this amounts to assignment of a malfunction of the brain and ocular cortex to "mere" dermatological citizenship.*

Additionally, in antithesis to auras, floaters have a kind of celebrity status, generating cocktail chatter, as if a middle-aged badge of honor. They are innocent, concrete, measurable objects, sometimes fixed and ineradicable; they last for years, usually the rest of people's lives. The sufferer may imagine he is seeing insects, phantom cars (while trying to look both ways at traffic lights), or other chimerical objects—so floaters are not trivial. Yet, by comparison, migraine auras are mysterious and transitory, scary, and difficult to gauge or qualify. People love to extol and complain about their charming

---

*See pages 153–155 for a further discussion of floaters.

floaters, while auras, as edgier and more disturbing traumas, occupy embargoed territory.

Fourth, the name "migraine aura" leads nowhere and means little, especially when medical research has provided virtually nothing regarding its cause or cure. One person experiences exotic but rare and brief distortions of vision; another has a condition called "migraine aura." Neither is understood, and neither is dangerous or cause for alarm. Additionally, neither can be treated. Of what practical use is the naming?

A fifth reason is, as noted earlier, the predominant connotation of the word "migraine" with a headache. When people hear that someone suffers a migraine, they think almost exclusively "cranial agony." Plus, almost anyone who sees an aura during or preceding severe cephalgia tends to emphasize the pain over the hallucination. This means that a large number of migraine-aura sufferers refer only to the "ouch" factor and cite the aura as the headache's mere disciple and forerunner.

Some call their auras "migraines" because that is more socially acceptable and elicits an appropriate response in a way that a description of weird visual distortions might not.

It is worth noting also that even many migraine headaches are often misdiagnosed as sinus headaches by sufferers: this mistake was made by 88 percent of 2991 patients in a 2004 study entitled "Prevalence of migraine in patients with a history of self-reported or physician-diagnosed 'Sinus' headache" by C. P. Schreiber and colleagues in an issue of the *Archives of Internal Medicine*.[107]

A sixth reason, the converse of the fifth, is that the identification of migraines with auras as expressions of the same underlying malady was not established until relatively recent times, so auras historically got classified with general hallucinations, trances, religious specters, psychoses, or other neurological disorders and did not develop their own line of testimony or literature. Auras have been "invisible symptoms," not only because of the later, more recent context imposed on them by migraine headaches but, prior to that (when they lacked migraine affiliation), because they had no consistent frame of reference at all.

A seventh explanation, touched on above, is: migraine auras are uncomfortable and disquieting, for they suggest what it is like to go blind or die. Real traumas, no matter how brief and select, retain a stubborn literalism, hammering at their own particulars until they create a private, isolated reality. They cannot be properly symbolized, cast in internal dialogues, or ameliorated by normal thought and social discussion, so their actual source vanishes into amnesia, and their elements become like a forgotten narrative of a multiple personality. Auras draw a blank because of either complete or partial traumatic dissociation. They are brief abductions generating instant gaps in memory.

Even regarding the facet that remains conscious, it is painful to ruminate on something so personal and distressing or to revive memories of it. Most sufferers do not wish to articulate tales of their auras or share their features with others. There also may be a premonition that mere discussion can set off an aura. Thinking about scotomata makes the eyes start to look for a fixation point, and then suddenly a suspicious glare or mottle can become a blind spot.

In any case, paradoxically, auras are neglected both because they are so trivial and incidental and so profound and frightening.

Eighth, by consequence of the above, auras tend to be normalized and minimized; their real nature is eradicated. Many people who have had them regularly from a young age find ways to cope with them silently, so their story doesn't enter into public discourse or even internal dialogue. The sense of startle or fear is diluted and replaced by mere annoyance or resignation. The event finds a mute role in commonplace reality even if it never becomes comfortable or normal. At least one doesn't have to go through denial each time that the landscape is coming apart.

I met an older man in the Oakland airport before a flight for which I had barely made it in time because of an earlier aura. As we began small talk, I brought up the events of my morning. He smiled and said, "I get auras like that once a week, but I ignore them. I just look around them like pulling aside a curtain with my mind."

A ninth, related reason why migraine auras are not part of everyday discourse is that people do not have *a way to talk about them*, either in social groups or families. Since scotomata are bizarre, indescribable, and incomprehensible, few sufferers develop a vocabulary that does the experience justice. A botched attempt to describe an aura might carry a taint of inadequacy or a stigma—as if one were taking drugs or loony—or it might simply fail to communicate the experience.

Our society does not provide many safe avenues for delving below the surface. People can prattle on about headaches, menstrual cramps, and even sexual fantasies more happily than about auras, which do not fit on the resumés of either ambitious careerists or worried conformists. In a culture in which "time is money"—and people on vacation or heading out from work are equally in a hurry to get somewhere for recreation—stopping on a dime for anything short of a heart attack or at least a splitting headache is not a popular option.

There is a premium on toughing it out, while there is a price to pay for being an invalid, even a temporary one. To yank yourself out of commission for temporary blindness suggests to others that you are sick or flawed, that you might black out at an unpredictable time. It elicits condescending sympathy or sick jokes: "Don't go Ray Charles on me." An ill-placed aura may impede professional advancement and damage reputation. After a commercial pilot told his superiors about a scotoma (an instance mentioned during a 2005 episode of the "Larry King Show" featuring migraines), he was fired.

For those suffering auras, exchanging narratives and comparing notes could be a form of mutual aid. Victims might reassure one another that, no matter how exotic the chimera forced on them, it is ordinary and common—others have seen the same displays, even in the same sequences.

It would not hurt, for instance, to be reminded in support groups that you can pull over to the roadside during an aura that starts while you are driving without having to worry about yourself as a candidate for forfeiture of your driving license. After all, if informal statistics are correct, at any one moment thousands of motor-vehicle operators in traffic throughout the world are hampered, even blinded, by scotomata—something at least to think about, even if it does not appear in the headlines with drunk driving and cell-phone distraction.

It would also be more comfortable to be able to announce during a meeting that you are undergoing an aura and need to be out of commission for about a half hour than to have to suffer in silence and potential ignominy for lapses in speech and judgment.

In summary, auras are ignored or avoided because of their brevity, harmlessness, lack of any explanation or context, traumatic amnesia, a paucity of cognitive and semantic concepts for them, fear of being regarded as inferior or damaged, unease that friends or colleagues will think one has a brain tumor or is going blind, a wish not to be the center of attention or to burden others, a capacity to work around a scotoma, and/or (despite any or all of the above) a general uncertainty about an aura's nature and consequences, even among those who have run the fire drill many times.

The First Migraine Aura and Later Incidence

Migraine auras can be both early-life phenomena that decrease in frequency with age and later-life phenomena that increase in frequency with age. The former pattern is, however, more common, with a subset being patients who start with classical migraines and lose the headache component during their thirties or forties but retain the auras. This confirms an underlying condition, deeper seated than any particular symptoms.

Migraine headaches tend to be chronic or recurrent in individuals and have a genetic history, inherited in classic Mendelian fashion. Studies of families have shown that the complex is inheritable on a recessive basis like sickle-cell anemia, with roughly 25–30 percent of offspring with one migrainous parent and 70–75 percent of those with both migrainous parents being migrainous too.[108] A dominant genetic locus, on the other hand, would lead to much higher inheritance rates. [I should add that these studies refer to classical or common migraines, not occasional naked auras (MAWOH).]

Migraine auras, when they are not experienced from early childhood throughout life, very often begin around the age of twenty, with clusters of new migraineurs in their thirties up to their fifties, and a few initial attacks occurring as late as people's nineties. Another "pattern" (noted above) is a single aura or a few auras—in childhood, from childhood through adolescence, or during adolescence—and then never again.

It is possible for anyone to have an isolated migraine aura without a headache at any time in life.

Chronic MAWOHs occur at all manner of intervals; among the more usual frequencies are: eight to ten times a year, once a month, and once a week. Usually people do not experience auras more than once a week. Other patterns are more disperse, with some people (as noted) experiencing gaps of years or decades between instances or clusters.

I have discovered puzzling patterns in my own aura cycles. At one point they went from fifteen in a year to twelve in the next year, to one, to nine, to fifteen, and back to nine. When I had only one in a period from 2002–2003, I thought that they might have stopped for good and was disappointed when the first one in a year occurred on exactly the same calendar day (July 4) as the one the previous year. The next one came sixty days later and was followed by two more, each thirty days after the previous one. Ninety-one days passed before the next and thirty days before the one after that. Perhaps the lunar cycle is one of many nonexclusive co-factors in migraines.

Whatever causes migraine auras in the first place, it should be noted that they often gain momentum. When one has occurred, the system tends to generate others, sometimes in clusters. When they occasionally end for good, after a number of episodes over years, they do so as inexplicably as they began.

Almost all migraine auras fall into the twenty- to thirty-minute category. However, in at least one instance mentioned on a medical Internet site, an intractable aura without a headache persisted for months and forced a patient into the hospital. I can no longer find that reference, but a 1998 Israeli study of reversal-of-vision metamorphopsia notes intermittent persistence of a transient optic cortical phenomenon for over a year.[109]

While collecting material for this book, I routinely asked people about auras and, if they experienced them, how they began. In one instance a woman described having her first in her early twenties. She was driving rather fast on a highway at the time and immediately panicked. Screeching to a halt and pulling onto the shoulder, she almost caused an accident. After the scotoma passed, she took the next exit and called her mother from a pay phone. "Why, that's a migraine," the flummoxed daughter heard. "We all get them in my family."

"I wondered why she never bothered to tell me. She told me everything else about her family and its foibles. I could have been killed!"

But this is in keeping with the mysterious "migraine aura silence."

Another woman *was* told about auras by her mother but, during her first attack, it took a moment to put two and two together: "I was driving to Tahoe when suddenly I have this visual stuff going on and I can't see the road. I think, 'Holy criminy, what is that?' I pull over, and then my migraine [headache] begins. I've always had migraines but never the auras. My mother gets the auras and used to talk about them, but I could never understand what she was seeing. Then suddenly I realized, 'This is that aura she's always talking about.' It was totally different than what I imagined from our conversations."

Cybernetic pioneer Marvin Minsky recalls his first two, very different auras (he had begun having common migraines a year or so earlier):

"One day, at age 17, I was walking alone at night during a snowstorm in a singularly quiet place. I noticed that the ground looked further away than usual, and then it seems that I was looking down from a height of perhaps 10 meters, watching myself crossing the field. . . .

"Another time, I forget the circumstances, I was looking at a tree and noticed that it was flickering strangely, sorta like a burning bush. In particular, I observed that it had acquired a sort of colorful, jagged, pulsating outline. 'My goodness,' I exclaimed to myself, 'it would seem that I'm experiencing a scintillating scotoma, and it looks just like the picture I remember from Duke Elder's *Textbook of Ophthalmology.* [Minsky's father was an ophthalmologist, and he had enjoyed perusing this book around the age of ten.] I'd better get ready for the migraine headache.' (I had had what seemed to be migraines before, but never with this phenomenon—which was rather gratifying because it confirmed an otherwise inconclusive diagnosis [e.g. the scotoma was validation he did not have a brain disease].) I always wondered if Moses (presuming that there ever was such a person) had migraines, too. Only a few such patients hear sounds as well."[110]

Other first instances I collected include the story of a fifty-one-year-old man passing from one hallway to another, en route from his office to attend a conference. As he enters the conference room, he feels it is not right and that something has been happening since he left his office. He can't see clearly and wonders what is blinding him. At first he thinks it is the fluorescent lighting and blinks, then closes, rubs, and reopens his eyes. The blot over the room is still there; in fact, it spreads and grows. Faces of people are divided in half. He struggles silently through the meeting, quite shaken.

One doctor had a few late-in-life-onset auras, and they all occurred along the same stretch of Highway 580 in Oakland. I tend to doubt that the landscape was the prime trigger but, in the context of co-factors, a particular scenery or, more likely, elicitation of migraine memory by a scenery, might be a proximal trigger. Auras, as we shall see, can be suggestive, slightly neurotic, and compulsive events.

A microbiologist described his first attack at the age of fifty: "I was driving my motorcycle. This was a Harley, and I was feeling pretty tough. Suddenly I couldn't read the license plate in front of me. I'd shift my head and it would be okay; then I couldn't read it again. Then a whole part of the landscape was missing, so I pulled over. I didn't feel so tough anymore."

The Onset of a Migraine Aura
and Its Common Circumstantial Triggers

Migraine arousal is implicit in the nervous system, and its co-factors either accumulate and discharge or are triggered by an event (or both). Migraines are often augured by incipient sensations, an undefined prodrome that may occur days, hours, or just minutes beforehand—premonitions that Sacks likens to seismic shock waves before an earthquake.[111]

A few people report a roaring sound, as of the sea heard in a shell, just before the appearance of phosphenes. Others feel persistent, strong tingling or a sensation of vibrating wires (paresthesias) in the feet, hands, face, and/or tongue areas where auras may occur, somewhat as if one were in contact with the sounding board of a piano.[112]

One migraineur recalls: "I seem to get a general upset of sensation all over the body. I especially notice the prickling in the fingers. . . . [T]hen the pain seems to rise from inside my skull and force its way outside my head. Then I get a throbbing in my ears where there was just prickling in my fingers, there's now a tingling sensation all over the place, even up my nose, as if I'd sniffed pepper or something like that."[113]

Sometimes an aura "rehearses" for days by propelling bright flickers or stars or luminous sparks across the field of vision.

Another migraineur says: "I know that something is happening to me, and I start to look around. I wonder if there is something the matter with the light. Then I notice that part of my visual field is missing."[114]

The pre-aura state can be one of uneasy excitement, ranging from a foreboding of "here comes that aura" to global disquiet or inap-

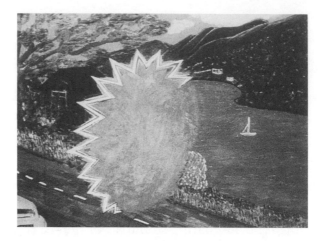

Figure 10: Scotoma with its scintillating edge surrounding a trailing blind spot, distorting an otherwise peaceful lake vista by a road (original in color). Obviously the emergence of a migraine aura makes driving difficult, for the driver can see nothing in the large inhibited zone. Migraine Art is reproduced by permission of the Migraine Action Association and Boheringer Ingelheim UK Limited.

propriate euphoria. Auras are sometimes preceded by manic, goofy, or inebriated sprees such that a normally safe driver speeds wildly, shouting and singing while he does, or a shy person goes around the house alternately yodeling and laughing.[115]

In an account from Sacks, a person riding a motorbike experienced a premonition of a migraine, so he got off; after a few minutes, he recounts, "I had an extraordinarily powerful tingling in my hands, nose, lips, and tongue. It seemed to be a continuation of the vibration of the motorbike, and at first I took this to be some simple after-effect." The vibrating extended into the fingers, the palms, then across his body. Finally his vision took up the sensation: "[A] feeling of motion was communicated to everything I saw, so that the trees, the grass, the clouds, etc., seemed to exhibit a silent boiling, to be quivering and streaming upwards in a sort of ecstasy. The hum of the crickets was all around me, and when I closed my eyes, this was immediately translated into a hum of color, which seemed to be the exact visual translation of the sound I heard."[116]

I will try to distinguish between generic and circumstantial triggers. Generic auras occur apparently because they are potentiated in the organism. Their basis may be a shift in biochemistry or a build-up of some sort of neural charge leading to a change in chemicoelectric status of some part of the brain. Generic auras are also influenced by diet, drugs, hormonal fluctuations (especially menstruation), missed sleep, sleep disorders of diverse sorts, "wrong" foods (but also skipped meals), overexertion, sinking barometric pressure, seasonal changes, sudden shifts in weather, air pollution, and perhaps astrobiological factors like phases of the Moon, sunspots, and (if we are to accept a scintilla of astrology) planetary alignments. Circumstantial auras arise from perceptual dissonance, compulsive activity, or cognitive dissociation. Of course, "generic" and "circumstantial" overlap, and it may make more sense to distinguish between environmental and purely neurological auras.

It should be no surprise that the most common circumstantial proprioceptive (as opposed to generic) trigger for migraine auras is light; to one degree or another most migraineurs are photosensitive. Sustained bright light and/or shifts of light and darkness encourage scotomata. Sacks indicts "crowded summer-beaches with sunlight beating down upon the ocean, and machine-shops blazing with unshielded lights."[117] Other photophobic triggers include a sudden glitter or brightness as off the rear window or bumper of a car in traffic, a glare from a window onto a TV monitor, a camera flash, the passage from a darker to more lit room (or *vice versa*), or the flickering light of certain frequencies such as a candle on a table in a darkened restaurant or a TV set that needs adjusting. Some scotoma-sufferers have had to have their television "repaired" to oscillate at a slightly different frequency—otherwise, they cannot watch their favorite shows without risking a fixation point. The flicker of a strobe is a particularly "effective" trigger; the scotoma loves the range of 8 to 12 stimuli per second, which replicates its own frequency.

For six months prior to my first ocular aura, a sustained flicker occasionally danced across the lower half of my field of vision, lasting anywhere from a few seconds to an hour. This palpitation was sometimes triggered by a passage between spaces of varying brightness but also by glares, reflections, and looking briefly at the sun. It was as though my iris had lost the capacity to adjust normally to changes in light, leading to a glimmering recoil. At least, so I imagined. Though not an aura, this was conceivably a gradual, long-term prodrome. I never saw it again after the auras began, though I did initially relate both effects to my decline in vision.

Sparkling, flickering, popping, and dancing of vitreous floaters, though not migrainous in themselves, may incite auras.

Cartoon figures, especially those in violent or madcap behavior, can provoke similar susceptibility.

Sudden, unexpected displacement in the visual field or moving scenery and shifting fields of objects from a vehicle may lead to part of the landscape getting tangled in its own patterns and becoming fixated. This speaks to the relationship between auras and motion sickness: each condition is provoked by a dissonance between an orientation for which the brain is prepared and an unexpected deviation from it (see pp. 117–119).

Auras can be aroused by sounds, by smells, tactilely, even from tastes (for instance, when all foods begin tasting the same or metallic). Sonophobic auras have been triggered by pneumatic drills; the irregular hum of traffic experienced from an upper-story window; heavy metal, rock, and rap music; flutes; crickets or frogs chirping at night; and the staccato but patterned din of a room full of people in separate conversations. In general, crowds, restaurants, theaters, and night-time bustle are migrainous. Dull, patterned drones like human chatter or shifts in the spectrum of crickets are more likely to provoke auras than mere loud noises like the amplified screech of the Rolling Stones or a car alarm in front of one's house.

A strong or unexpected odor or "off" taste or aftertaste may convert into an aura. Something in the sensation causes the neural process to trip over its own feedback, using the aroma or flavor as its fixation.

Possible triggers are as treacherous and limitless as the ways Orpheus was duped into looking at Eurydice after the gods forbade him her sight. These may be as specific and unusual as the glimpsing of a set of Venetian blinds with its sharp alternations of slats and openings, the wind moving curtains, fingers passing before the eyes, a striped shirt across a room, floral designs on wallpaper, or an Oriental rug. A reported migraine began when the surface of the wallpaper shimmered like the surface of a pond.[118]

The inciting flutter can be as minor as a digital clock changing a character, a fly suddenly alighting (or even stopping its movement after landing), shade imposed by a moving cloud, the blur of a darting bird, or a paper blowing past peripheral vision. It merely has to be noticed in a certain way to be migraine-inducing.

Other peculiar instigators in migraine literature include a cubist painting in a museum, an Escher drawing in a book, a typographical error in an article, a momentary confusion about what one is looking at such that an object changes definition or is perceived as something else much closer or further away, or a sudden reversal of foreground and background as in an optical illusion.

One patient of Sacks describes especially devious etiologies: "Some [of my migraines] may be provoked by unexpected twists and oddities which suddenly strike me. A button may be done up askew in a coat. The whole coat looks askew and bothers me oddly. Then this skew in the coat *becomes* a skew or twist in my vision, sets off a local distortion in my visual field, which may then spread until it engulfs the greater part of the visual field. Or it may be something askew in a face—like a tic, or a grimace, or spasm—some asymmetry. Once it was set off by seeing a man with Bell's Palsy. The perception is momentary, but it can set off a spatial disturbance that can last for several minutes."[119]

Perhaps the most powerful instigator of migraine auras is previous auras. It seems once the cortex "knows" or remembers prior attacks, it responds to not only discharges from within the brain—the likely base cause of migraines—but migrainously evocative images, sounds, and sensations that suggest an aura.

Some individuals may incite their own auras by staring overhard at spots, boundaries of objects, blurred objects, or contrasting zones of light. During periods of susceptibility, it is relatively easy to provoke a new aura by paralyzed attention to glares, oscillations, or peripheral movements. Even the thought of what a migraine aura is like can trigger one, so this discussion may provoke a few readers. During periods of unaccountable migraine immunity, one can react more casually without risking fixation. However, one doesn't always know when he or she has entered a new regime of susceptibility.

Sacks remarks that "the entire migraine may be perpetuated by one or another of its own symptoms." A resonance within the migraine template—a scotoma memory, as it were—becomes its own self-initiating cause: auras are habit-forming. "In short ... a *migraine can become a response to itself.* Given the initial provocation, the original impetus, one may envisage that the subsequent continuance of many migraines may arise in this fashion from a series of self-perpetuating internal drives—a positive feed-back—so that the entire reaction is bound within its own circularity."[120] However neurologically chasmal the cerebral discharge, once loaded into the system it can be dischraged by a mere recollection or aggravation.

This obsessive aspect of migraine magnifies distinctions that would be absorbed or subsumed if an image were not attached to so trenchantly. The patterning of an external anomaly locks into and elicits a latent reverberation. The commitment may be as biologically fixed as a tic but, because it enlists cognition, it operates through the psyche. In auras (as opposed to phobias) the compulsive aspect is neural more than neurotic, but that doesn't mean there is no neurotic component. So while auras are more spastic than neuroses, they are more psychological than many spasms.

The bound energy and discharge of some auras may be similar to that of certain panic attacks wherein a person responds not so much to a dreaded event as to a compulsive fixation or apprehension of such an event, which invokes latent anxiety. In that fashion, concern about an impending migraine aura (because one has had them before) is a vexing factor that can turn an otherwise-innocent symptom, like an askew button, into a co-factor in relation to some unresolved fantasy or defense mechanism. The mind, not the button, is the cue, as it refuses to allow the anomaly to pass, instead disorganizing it into an askew universe.

The Relation of Auras to Vision

Bleary or uncertain sight is a circumstantial cause of migraine auras. Blurs can originate either generically from near- and far-sightedness and astigmatism or secondarily via acts of staring and straining to see, and they have a spasmodic, self-enhancingly migrainous quality. If this prognosis is accurate, a certain percentage of the population began experiencing migraine auras (like me) at approximately the time their vision developed age-related deficiencies.* This doesn't mean that "vision" is the sole or even primary cause of auras, but it

---

*Some vision educators believe that stress rather than age is the cause.

can be a significant co-factor that tips events in the cortex in a migrainous direction. At least that is my hypothesis.

In this scenario, there is a latent focusing device that organizes streams of ocular synapses flowing into the mind and processes the visual substrate. As it begins chronically to lose acuity, it gets stressed and recalibrates itself. A person starts seeing unexpected fuzzinesses and is not able to resolve certain patterns into recognizable objects or cannot read print that he or she formerly could scan at will. When one strains to see a figure within a blur, at a certain point traffic in the ocular apparatus becomes anomalous and creates an artifact to distribute the dissonance.

Just as the brain is ever organizing stimuli and information into usable and functional patterns, it can also lapse into asynchrony and begin disorganizing data and patterns. In such a regime a simple anomaly (that most of the time would be overridden or minimized by dominant organizing patterns in the brain/neural hierarchy) becomes focalized, magnified, and fixated.*

Between the mind's seeing a double or indistinct figure and its expectation to be able to focus clearly, there arises a phantom thing that is neither the blur nor a lucid image but a gestalt of the two. As the contradiction becomes more discordant than the feedback loop between sensation and proprioception can sustain, a proxy landscape replaces the real one. Objects change character in the mind; figure and ground reverse such that what seemed to be inside the field of one thing becomes the periphery of another; cues for distance, scale, and size lose their reference points, while relationships of boundary and parallax flutter. Letters become not only blurs in the eye but hieroglyphs in the brain. At some point in this circularity, a real aura may manifest, a cumulative amorphism that becomes self-reinforcing, and this propagates a tiny, transiently indelible mot-

---

*For the application of chaos theory to migraine auras, see pp. 141–146.

tle. Perception has already created the replica of a scotoma, so the mind then "convinces" the brain to turn it into an actual one.

For example, a person rightly anticipates human faces in a crowd but instead is shown an elephant head or blank face on a human body. This elicits a "correction." The oddity caused by strained vision—e.g. an indistinct, uninterpretable pattern or a grotesque thing the mind knows can't be real—becomes a different kind of distortion, an abstract, contentless myth or fairy tale that must wind through its entire cycle before the visioning apparatus of eye and mind-brain can restore prior lucidity. This might also be vision's utility function, its attempt to repair itself (see pp. 128–130).

In summary, an aura is a relic that is sometimes biological and then perceptual, sometimes perceptual and then biological, sometimes both more or less simultaneously, and always bound within the circularity of its own resonance. It is not only a shift in the chemistry and physiology of the brain; it is a preconscious gnarl in perception itself, a mirage or hybrid that is so convincing and confusing to the image-comprehending aspect of the mind that it produces a lasting figment, a paroxysm with enduring sensory effects. That is why a scotoma does not operate as a passing optical illusion or mistaken identity that dissipates as soon as it is recognized—it is a confusion that imprints itself into a neural cycle that then must have its own endemic expression and meaning.

Of course, all of these same processes occur in people with 20/20 eyesight, including very young people, and thus are not necessarily a symptom or precursor of visual deterioration. With or without vision problems, one can elicit a migrainous aura—in the presence of co-factors—by staring, which inherently causes an image to become migrainous. Not only does one not see very well while staring, but persistent fixations rigidify the ocular, cranial, and cervical muscles while reinforcing stressful neuromuscular habits. Educators in the Bates Method and kindred systems for vision improvement train pupils not to fixate but instead to keep moving the focal point (e.g. brushing objects with an imaginary pencil or feather attached to one's nose), breathing deeply, and blinking regularly (see footnote on p. 209).

Only if one stares chronically does everyday vision get blurrier with time. Thus, any long-term deleterious effect of auras on eyesight is probably a secondary consequence of a person becoming so mistrustful of his/her vision that s/he begins fixating compulsively to stave off auras. "I had 2 auras in the past 2 days, after not having any for maybe 5 or 6 years…," writes Cather in the halfbakery chatroom. "Now am paranoid of getting them all the time."[121] When one becomes hyper-watchful, walking on eggshells, subject to ocular fits and starts, scotomata can shape phobic and/or obsessive personalities, while continuing to worsen vision. A migraine aura becomes a migraine neurosis.

If you are stuck in such a pattern, try to restore confidence and relaxation in your sight; don't stare or strain to resolve blurs; let them resolve themselves gracefully: if a migraine aura comes, it comes, but don't maintain a vigil against it.

Psychosomatic Factors

Insofar as auras (like dreams) raise internal events to the status of real experiences while marginalizing the external world, some of their dynamics and imagery draw on a realm of emotional compensations and projections. The affective component of migraines is not only varied and subtle but has paradoxical elements. Pure anger has been known to trigger an aura, as rage sublimates into a scotoma. The migraine attack then represents another kind of attack on the target in the world, projected (as it were) inward. Repeated tension with a partner (personal or professional) can lead to an aura either during or, more commonly, just after the peak of a stressful encounter. Suppressed rage and fake easy-goingness may also be migraine co-factors.

Yet elation and a sense of triumph may likewise propagate a scotoma, almost as if guilt from success generated sensory depression, or a heightened emotion self-transformed into dullness and fatigue. The fluctuating boundaries and thresholds between pleasure and pain, joy and grief, anger and suppressed anger, happiness and irritable excitation, fun and a headache—especially when an element of shame and self-criticism is incorporated—can beget unstable psychosomatic landscapes in which migraines develop.

One trigger to auras is a state of agitated and anticipatory excitement when too much is happening at once—the start of a party a person is hosting, simultaneous with receiving an important telephone call, simultaneous with a great idea to try out at work. At a certain point, none of these excitements is particularly exciting anymore. They have combined to produce a deadening, empty effect, like a delicious meal turning tasteless in the mouth (also a migrainous effect). In the trough of sensation that follows, a dot begins oscillating. The ensuing scotoma derails the prickly mood so that, by the time it has dissolved, a charged irritability has mutated into a calmer, more balanced state.

Euphoric and choleric etiologies of auras represent different levels of the same reality, and they both present opportunities for emotional metamorphosis and personal growth but also can trigger depression, anxiety, and other despondent states.

Some auras also bear aspects of "reaction formation," e.g. the sufferer uses migraines to protect himself/herself against forbidden impulses and fantasies when other defenses and repressions are inadequate. In that case, the migraine is preferable to, for instance, a negative projection onto a loved one out of vexation or resentment or from some neurotic requisite. If a scotoma emerges in a loop in which it is diametrically opposed to tabooed desires or hostile "wishes," it can serve as a mechanism of ego-reinforcement and control.

Migraines and their auras have similarly been set off by both somatic events and their cessation. Phases in menstrual cycles, menstruation itself, allergic attacks, constipation, a physical aggravation, and injurious accidents are all migraine elicitors. Any of these conditions may inversely produce a replacement cycle with migraines and auras such that migraines *do not occur* when they do; e.g. auras appear almost exclusively during periods of no allergies or regular bowel movements and cease during bouts of allergic attack or constipation.[122]

These malaises may be analogous events or have analogous elements to migraines such that they either synergize with them or replace them in neurosomatic homeostases. For instance, a person who is injury-prone and also a migraine sufferer may not experience migraines at all during periods of frequent accidents (and *vice versa*). Migraines can also be supplanted by epilepsy (see p. 115).

Replacement cycles suggest an underlying guilt or an unresolved neurosis (likely at an unconscious level) driving both events such that migraines serve a compensatory function. They can occur *instead of* other physical or psychological symptoms and conversely be subrogated by them. The neurosis does not cause or "cure" the migraine but, depending on its reciprocal co-factor, either stimulates or dampens the symptoms' energetic basis.

A migraine may itself be a homeostatic mechanism, bringing extreme ranges of emotions and psychosomatic conditions into balance and providing an alternate to self-destructive guilt. (That does not mean that the same substitutions could not be propelled by exclusively physiological or hormonal factors, though it is hard to imagine a migraine without some psychosomatic co-factor.)

Sacks reports on an Auschwitz inmate who was imprisoned for six hellish years in a concentration camp, during which his wife, parents, and all his close relatives were murdered, yet he suffered no migraines in that period despite his previous proclivity for them. After he was freed, he began having more than weekly attacks. Sacks remarks that migraines would have been "lethally maladaptive" in the concentration camp but made sense in the context of survivor's guilt and depression afterwards.[123]

This holocaust survivor's attacks also waned during streaks of injury from accident-proneness as well as during psychotic depressions, indicating that when he was starting to feel "better" or tolerated functioning in his new life, he was overtaken by migraine sensitivity. Once again, migraines do not so much have a set meaning as retrieve old traumas and shadow selves and bring opposites into balance. That is why they can embody contradictory contents.

"Coming after the storm" is a migraine hallmark. When one is performing on stage, lecturing, taking an exam, negotiating a deal, giving birth, shooting a movie, flying a plane, fighting in battle, robbing a bank, conducting courtship, making love, pregnant (even women who suffer chronic migraines otherwise), migraines rarely occur—but *after* a major event, when the period of engagement, heightened activity, heroism, and excitation has passed, the migraines start again. "It's not a stress thing," one woman commented; "It's only when I relax that I get the migraine."

Whether this represents a subliminally intentional delay of the symptom in order to prevent its interference with something important (as with the genocide survivor) or the natural attraction of migraines to post-excitement valleys, or both, is impossible to know. Either way, migraines resemble other fugues, dumb stupors, and hangovers that nurture recuperation and bursts of new energy.

A common cycle is weekend-only migraines. Many people get migraines uniquely on weekends or rarely at other times. This would suggest the tendency for a migraine to embody, on a level of cognitive-biological feedback, rebound from periods of exertion and over-activity. Else, how would the cells and molecules know it was a Sunday?

Aspects of migraines that recognize personality structure in this way are fabricated primordially much as the human organism concocts dreams, works of art, neuroses, and symbols—by sublimation, transference, displacement, and reaction formation.

Dreams

Auras may begin during sleep and elapse entirely in a dream—a pulsing light or oscillating feature in the dreamed landscape blossoms into a scotoma. The flickering may originate in any number of dream components: blinking traffic lights, an unnaturally gleaming airplane, or scenery itself commencing to wobble. The dreamer, if she awakens at this point, does so into a full-blown aura.

In a dream I am attending a seminar and following a lecturer's presentation on the blackboard. Then I can't read the chalk marks and, even though dreaming, begin to worry that a migraine aura might begin. While straining to make out the letters, I notice a flashing spot. I wake and am relieved it is just a dream ... only to see a "real" scintillating scotoma against the window.*

Usually one gets to escape such hallucinations by waking up, but migraines can merge with dreamscapes while retaining autonomous identities; they don't always sublimate. While the same can transpire with other physiological components (digestive upset, diverse

---

*This dream is my own.

aches or pains, and genital excitation), for the most part these convert into elements of the dream. Their metamorphosis, declared Sigmund Freud, protects the oneirological process in its task of symbolic translation, e.g. to keep the dreamer safely asleep. Scotomata, however, tend to remain scotomata, and the dream adapts to their identity as such.

Migraine auras are comparable but not equivalent to dreams in that they don't suffuse the mind with an illusory symbolized world or work out complicated emotional puzzles through proxies and aliases; they contain enough fixed biological elements so as *not* to be able to transmute elaborate psychological nuances. Yet, in their own primitive and incomplete fashion, they receive, condense, and metabolize feelings and unresolved issues, and process pseudolibidinal charges, resistance, and projections.

While migraine is similar to other primitive psychosymbolic modes of conversion in its uses of preexisting cathexes and latent traumas to make new material with altered potential, it is also individual, almost unique, in the way in which it displaces neurotic and psychotic elements into brief proprioceptive dramas of survival, identity, and reality.

Migraine auras are psychosomatically like dreams in that they express uncompensated contents of the psyche and gaps in the body's neurohormonal equilibrium. If they are suppressed, even as when a person is sleep deprived and cannot dream, substitute symptoms arise in their stead and exact a cost from both emotions and organs. Dreams and auras each heal as well as distort, "maim" as well as cure.

The literal explicitness of an aura in a dream gives us a clue as to its nature—it doesn't assimilate into anything but a dreamed aura; it coincides with an oneirological narrative identically to how it fits into waking perception. This suggests a set psychosomatic relationship between auras and the cerebral process, perhaps at the core of the invertebrate brain.*

It is possible that at least some of the hallucinated components and image-streams of third-stage migraines may be interpretable at multiple levels in the way that dreams are, as expressions of instincts, conflicts, or archetypes. This would not invalidate their purely anatomical derivation but would mean that, like dreams, they embody secondary paradigms related to emotional charge and waking function.

A dreamlike aspect of auras is revealed in chatrooms whenever the opportunity to exchange accounts has an effect on dialoguers' migraines. At one point, for instance, Sarenka writes: "I'm not sure why, but since ... reading about everyone else's different aura descriptions, mine have suddenly become more varied in certain ways. This morning I had one that I swear had some coloring to it for a while, even though I'd never had colored ones before."[124]

Though this is not typical transference, apparently migraines can "learn" from ordinary language and translate both conscious and preconscious components into sensory ones. This suggests that auras have something more at their base than the raw excitations that characterize other seizures and neural excitations; they are, at least in part, psychosomatic and symbolizing phenomena.

---

*A dreamer can produce alias "auras" too—ones that dissolve with the rest of the oneirology at waking—but such nonmigrainous replicas are a different kettle of fish as, at times, elements of the dreamwork hatch a fictive "scotoma" to represent—not *be*—some aspect of inner conflict or resistance to a suppressed feeling.

Thus, while auras are *not* dreams or libidinal events in their reduced capacity for symbolism, they may carry a different, phylogenetic and recuperative symbolism and a protolibidinal eros. The symbolic representation of the migraineur's psychological and even archetypal state might be inscribed in the vegetative components of the scotoma and its motifs.

Auras might be considered brief dream equivalents in that both migraines and scotomata function as homeostatic triggers at the level of the brainstem, e.g. a lizard stage of consciousness emerging out of piscean unconsciousness, alertness out of paroxysm, otherness out of ego. A distinction between dreams and scotomata implies a recognition that oneself is a discrete entity, separate from objects and sensations. In humans, millennia after the primitive psychosomatic correlation between ego and object, auras perform more as "failed dreams" insofar as our primitive oneirogenic vibrations have evolved into full extraliminal trances with emotional and archetypal contents—elaborate fugues that can be pleasurable and enchanting—whereas our atavistic migrainoid bursts have devolved into basically optical headaches.*

The Resolution of a Migraine Aura

Fortunately, migraine auras do not have to be treated medically for them to end. They resolve by running their natural course. The aura eventually crosses beyond visibility or dissipates, usually far sooner than the mayhem it stirs up would intimate.

Not only do auras (and ensuing headaches) culminate spontaneously but their abatement is often accompanied by a variety of soothing and/or invigorating, purgative, and cleansing events. Dissolution may give rise to an outburst of tears, copious urination, a

---

* I will continue to speculate on this topic later (see pp. 131-139).

bowel movement, a fit of irrepressible sneezing, a discharge of sweat glands throughout the body, a nosebleed, or a running nose.

A deep and restorative post-migraine sleep sends many sufferers into a realm beyond life, full of epiphanies, fleeting insights, a sense of incredible solutions for thorny problems looming just up ahead. People feel a surge of energy with revivification of their whole system, a profound calm and euphoria not unlike the euphoria at the beginning of some attacks—a conviction that all has been suddenly made right with the world. Sacks refers to "the sense of extreme refreshment, and almost of rebirth.... Such states do not represent a mere restoration to the pre-migraine condition, but a swing in the direction of arousal, a *rebound* after the migrainous trough."[125] Edward Liveing, writing under the nineteenth-century rubric "*on megrim, sick-headache, some allied disorders, and the pathology of nerve-storms,*" concluded: "[the patient] awakes a different being."[126]

A 55-year-old man, quite pleased with his migraines, reports, "There is a greater depth and speed and acuity of thought.... I keep recalling things long forgotten, visions of earlier years will spring to mind." His wife, however, complains, "He walks back and forth, talks in a repetitive manner in a sort of monotone; he seems to be in a trance...."[127]

Hildegard of Bingen praised her favorite aura thusly: "[W]hen I look upon it, every sadness and pain vanishes from my memory, so that I am again as a simple maid and not as an old woman."[128]

Many migraineurs conversely experience global disorientation and/or fear after the aura has passed. The discomfort can be as straightforward as an apprehension that scotomata will never stop, turning into an unrelieved series of flashing spots in a cyclonic sea. Because the basic coherence of the visual field has been challenged and undermined, congruity does not just immediately return. A person may feel uneasy for quite a while (hours, days, even weeks afterwards) that a new aura is about to begin. Thus, as noted earlier, daily activity and vision are compromised.

Even without heightened apprehension, the visual field after the passage of a scotoma may remain skittery, unstable, shimmering, flattened, punctuated by lingering stars and brief gaps, perhaps vibrating and shaky in spots (as when looking at areas of high contrast, borders between three-dimensional objects, and/or shadowed landscapes). Or, more to the point, ordinary brief flutters and normal artifacts and spasms of vision that quickly could be adjusted or dismissed prior to auras become chronic and persistent. Every afterimage, glare, floater, and optic sizzle becomes suspicious. It looks ripe for fixation.

Vision itself is not perfect, even under ideal circumstances, but for everyday sight the mind tends to override ordinary dissonances and moiré-like effects created by lines, areas of contrast, and the mundane procession of textured, complicated patterns flowing in relationship to one another. The eyes, neural synapses, and brain collaborate moment to moment in presenting a cleaned, corrected "video" to the mind. However, once a migraine aura splashes into that, sending its ripples through landscapes and objects, it not only shatters the immaculate streaming of visual designs at that moment; it permanently snaps the innocent illusion of pure vision and teaches the mind to see its own familiar gestalt as an imperfect rendition of an unsteady, pointillistic reality.

A person who develops anxieties in relation to migraine auras and, after an aura or during the genesis of a chronic migraine condition, unconsciously transfers stresses from life into the visual field, may gradually begin to notice many more of the little glitches and corruptions of ordinary sight, to the point of compulsively observing and enhancing them. The visual compulsion persists even when he or she is not suffering an aura. Soon a mild hallucination develops such that the landscape seems to be continuously shimmering or spasming in spots or skipping across its patterns. After all, vision tends to be the first sense to unravel when people take mind-altering drugs or undergo ecstatic reveries or panic attacks. "Seeing things" is a complement to diverse psychological, psychopathological, and psychospiritual states.

During an aura cycle in 2003 I began to see the living room in our summer house as liquid and pulsating. Upon awakening one night from an anxious dream, I went downstairs and turned on the light to reveal a scenery throbbing and undulating. I was so concerned about my vision that I momentarily panicked and for at least a minute did not realize that smoke had backed up from the woodstove and was densely pouring out. My state of disorientation was such that my sense of smell had to tell my sight what it was actually seeing.

My experience is also that a scotoma doesn't just slide off the edge of the visual field like a stick rolling over a waterfall; it turns intermittent at the periphery of sight, coming and going for a while, and then, once it is mostly gone, objects everywhere remain a little flickery or quavery with tiny spasms like twitches, usually on their edges. They may also present a vague enigmatic sightlessness, as if they can't be seen even though they can. That is, the negative scotoma feels as though it is still there but, when interrogated visually, each thing in turn is accounted for, nothing is missing. Yet objects still have to be looked at multiple times, scanned at different angles, and identified individually, to be declared safely out of a lurking blind spot (see Lashley's account of perplexing blank areas on p. 39).

Some people experience full hallucinations or dysphasia after scotomata have passed and, like those having psychotic breakdowns, do not grasp immediately that they are experiencing:

"A very strange thing happened, shortly after my vision came back. First, I couldn't think where I was, and then I suddenly realized that I was back in California. . . . It was a hot summer day. I saw my wife moving about on the verandah, and I called her to bring me a Coke. She turned to me with an odd look on her face, and said, 'Are you sick or something?' I suddenly realized that it was a winter's day in New York, that there was no verandah, and that it wasn't my wife but my secretary who was standing in the office looking strangely at me."[129]

There is a tendency for chronic migraineurs never to completely recover and thus to develop fully migrainous personalities, in a state of continual uncertainty as to whether they are just completing a migraine, about to begin one, or are having one at a subperceptual level. Is an object missing, or was it actually moved—or was there no object there in the first place? This becomes its own quasi-autistic, semi-dyslexic lifestyle. Sacks refers to patients who live "in a half-space, a half-universe . . . their consciousness has been reorganized, and they do not know it."[130] Great art and literature have emerged from such states, in part as an urgent attempt to heal what has been injured.

Siri Hustvedt, who has woven a migraine aesthetic into her novels, recalls a dramatic tactile aura that encompassed both transference and rebirth shadowing her wedding. In a striking example of a migraine tempering elation, she was literally tugged into her new identity: "I was married at twenty-seven in June of 1982 and spent my honeymoon in Paris with my new husband. One afternoon, we were in the Gallerie Maeght. My husband had left me for a few moments, and as I stood there alone, I felt what I think was my left arm (but it may have been my right) yanked by some invisible force into the air. This ghost then threw me backward and slammed me into the wall. It lasted only seconds. I recovered entirely, but when I stepped into the street with my husband, I looked at the buildings and pedestrians and had the curious feeling that my eyesight had suddenly improved, that I was seeing with a new clarity and sharpness, and then a feeling of elation arrived. 'I have never been so happy in my life,' I said to myself."

Nonetheless, the cycle had not completed itself: "The headache arrived later in the day...."[131]

Russian novelist Fyodor Dostoyevsky regarded one of his likely epileptic auras not as a pathology but an epiphany: "There are moments, and it is only a matter of five or six seconds, when you feel the presence of the eternal harmony...a terrible thing is the frightful clearness with which it manifests itself and the rapture with which it fills you. If this state were to last more than five seconds, the soul could not endure it and would have to disappear. During these five seconds I live a whole human existence, and for that I would give up my whole life and not think that I was paying too dearly."[132]

Tribulation is a handmaiden to personal growth, not only because a transformative experience challenges categories of body and self but because a person is also resisting or repressing a new way of self-organizing—after all, a force that is initiating even beneficial change is perceived as a threat or incursion. In truth, most events can be used for either good or ill, for advancement or retrenchment. The experience and its interpretation lie in the beholder and are not by any means absolute. An open wound can be a gateway to inner life. Whether an outcome is therapeutic or detrimental may depend on the person and his or her receptivity at the time. In Buddhist meditation, for instance, the state of emptiness (*sunyata*) associated with enlightenment can be horrific and terrifying to a person who is not ready to experience that level of reality.

By that measure, migraine auras are an opportunity to be reborn—happier and more whole with a fuller appreciation of existence. This is the unexpected gift of autonomous psychospiritual processes, even ones arising from the body: they make the world over and increase awareness. This is probably a better way of experiencing an aura than dread, victimization, or pretending that nothing is happening.

Once we make our peace with migraine auras, we may find that our experience of them becomes invested with meanings and bounties we did not foresee. It is not important to know whether these reside in the auras themselves or are the inevitable result of witnessing the world with receptivity and love.

Whatever they are, auras are profound neuropsychic events, and the aspects of them that are most disturbing and uncomfortable may contain the richest opportunities for understanding and inner transformation.

The Nature and Meaning of Migraine Auras: Their Deeper Phenomenology

A scotoma takes away not only part of the vision field, but its innate cohesion. When scenery is punctured by flashing sawteeth imposing figments and artifacts on it and/or fracturing it into independent zones or mosaics, the scotoma interferes at a fundamental level with the way in which the brain constructs meaning. While some people experience mainly a landscape through broken glass, others notice a more fundamental disaffiliation such that, not only is the physiology of vision fragmented, but the gist and meaning of one part of it are not connected to the other. Insofar as the basis of self is located in a personal body extending in space and time and kinesthetic continuity, suddenly one's basic identity and humanity are at stake.

People sometimes turn their heads to assure themselves that objects still exist in their original places. They may move a candlestick, salt-shaker, or chair to warrant that the landscape behind it continues in the expected way—that the object does not cover a hole in reality.

Sacks recalls a patient who, during the passage of a scotoma, was able to tell time on his watch only by looking first at the minute or hour hand and then at the other and then at each number, one by one, and gradually puzzling out their collective meaning. The watch by itself was a blind spot and a blur.[133] This disjunction, not unlike that of the man who mistook his wife for a hat, shows how optic meaning as well as ocular perception is affected. The aura hits at the core of how location, distance, and sequence are labeled in the nervous system.

The distortion may be even subtler: there may be no perceptible dissociation of the actual landscape—things look deceptively normal, appear exactly as they always did, but do not feel right, do not seem themselves; they have become unstable and at any moment might erode. This could be because they have developed a faint oscillation or look stale and plain, too ordinary and two-dimensional to be real, especially by comparison to the complexly manifesting, fiery scotoma which is nowhere or creates its own geography.

The schism is *not* ocular but in the brain itself. The flashing mottle and blind spot declare themselves directly to the cortex without the intervention of sensation or language; they tell us that they are *more* real than the world itself, or at least more primary and indelible. Outside the arena of language and symbolic mediation, auras cannot be fought off intellectually.

Normal experiencing of reality ceases too, not only in the present when it is happening, but in the past (which no longer makes sense and may seep into the "now" as *déjà vu*) and the future (which has been ruined and can no longer happen, for regular time has terminated and been replaced by migraine time). As the tags of human context crumble, scotomata cease to be simple interruptions of vision and enter into an eidetic realm.

A scotoma may pass in a matter of minutes, but the ego-self observes it in horror because it is altering consciousness in a way that it is powerless to stop.[134] Apprehension ranges from borderline alarm and concern to abject terror and premonition of death. The migraineur undergoes in a very immediate way a perception that scientists and philosophers arrive at analytically. Far from being automatic or guaranteed, "the spacetime continuum [is something] which the patient with migraine both suffers and creates."[135]

A psychoanalyst who, in the course of his professional routine, treated all manner of anxiety, panic, and psychosis, was troubled in a baffling way by his own migraine auras. He experienced them two or three times a year since early childhood, more often than not succeeded by headaches:

"I may be seeing as a patient someone I know well, sitting across the desk, with my gaze fixed upon them. Suddenly I become aware that something is wrong—although at this point I cannot say what it is. It is a sense of something *fundamentally* wrong—something impossible and contrary to the order of nature.

"Then I suddenly 'realize'—*part of the patient's face is missing:* part of their nose, or their cheek, or perhaps the left ear. Although I continue to listen and speak, my gaze seems transfixed—I cannot move my head—and a sense of horror, of the impossible, steals over me. The disappearance continues—usually until half the face has disappeared and, with this, that same half of the room. I feel paralyzed and petrified in some sort of way. It never occurs to me that something is happening to my vision—I feel something incredible is happening in the *world.* It doesn't occur to me to 'check' on the existence of what seems to be missing. It never occurs to me that I am having a migraine, even though I have had the experience dozens of times before...."

This common response to onset (usually not so well articulated) provides us with two hints: First, the aura does not carry the intrinsic message that it is a migraine, so the initial reaction is that the hallucination is a real thing—despite the fact its predecessors have visited many times before and have always proven to be a mirage. Second, people with chronic migraines lose track of when one is happening, even as they lose track of time and language. They do not know if something is actually missing—erased by a brief optical illusion, glare, blind spot, etc.—or if it is "scotoma-blotted-out," carrying deficits beyond hallucination. Isn't it remarkable that, despite so many previous episodes and profound psychiatric knowledge, this migraineur still feels that he is experiencing a real event rather than a neural artifact?

"I don't exactly feel that anything is 'missing,' but I fall into a ridiculous, obsessive doubt. I seem to lose the *idea* of a face; I 'forget' how faces look—something happens to my imagination, my memory, my thinking.... It is not that half the world mysteriously 'disappears,' but that I find myself in doubt as to whether it was ever there. There seems to be a sort of hole in my memory and mind and, so to speak, a hole in the world; and yet I cannot imagine what might go in the hole. There is a hole and there isn't a hole—my mind is utterly confounded. I have the feeling that my body—that *bodies* are unstable, that they may come apart and lose parts of themselves—an eye, a limb, amputation—that something vital has disappeared, but disappeared *without trace,* that it has disappeared *along with the 'place' it once occupied.* The horrible feeling is of nothingness nowhere."

Gradually he realizes that he is having an aura and that this has happened before. "[A]n immense sense of relief floods over me...."

"But even knowing this does not *correct* the perception.... There is still a certain residue of dread, and a fear that the scotoma may go on forever."[136]

He adds that he is never so afraid of anything else.

In an equally unsettling account, Sacks describes a woman who experiences that the left side of her body totally disappears, leaving nothing, just a blank, concomitant with the blank in her visual field. This reads to her as a blank in the universe, and she feels an inconsolable cosmic terror, as though nothing will ever be right again. Her intuition is that the hole "is like death, and that one day it will get so large that it will 'swallow' her completely."[137]

The blind spot is literally as well as archetypally a "shadow." It is a crack in nature and a warning that the crack may ultimately establish primacy, swallow up creation from within, and become more real than it. Hustvedt explores this nihilistic aspect through a character in her novel *The Blindfold*:

"The image was changing. With more curiosity than alarm, I noticed a small black hole in the face. How can that be? I said to myself. It wasn't there before. But not for a moment did I doubt its reality. The hole grew, eating away the left eye and nose, and then the dread came, cold and absolute, a terror so profound it created a kind of paralysis. I was transfixed. The hole was devouring the entire image, the face and hair, the shoulders, breasts, and torso, and I saw only the arm stumps hanging there alone for an instant, and then they too were engulfed, but like a person in a dream, I couldn't cry out. There was no sound in me, and I watched as the hole began to swallow the picture frame."

As the character's vision returns to "normal," reality doesn't: "[Objects] came into focus slowly—blurry, nameless things from another world. I heard breathing and thought that there was someone else in the room before I realized it was my own respiration, loud and uneven like an invalid's. The room returned to itself, and I saw the photograph lying facedown on the floor, an insignificant white rectangle.

"It was over, and I could feel pain in my head. I suffer from migraine and am susceptible to nervous ticks and minor hallucinations, but I have never been able to write off these experiences as aberrations that are purely neurological, because while they are happening, I am convinced that I am seeing the truth, that the terrible fragility and absence I feel is the world—stark and unclothed. That nakedness is irretrievable. It is left behind in the raw, voiceless place that exists beyond the muttering dreams of everyday life, where you cannot ask to go but must be taken."[138]

Later this character recounts a migraine aura to her doctor, recalling one of the author's (see p. 89):

"[A]s soon as I stepped inside my apartment, I felt a tug on my left arm, just as if someone had yanked it hard. I lost my balance and fell down. I was so dizzy and sick to my stomach that I didn't get up for a long time. While I was sitting there on the floor, I saw lights, hundreds of bright sparks that filled up half the room, and after they disappeared, I saw a big, ragged hole in the wall. That hole scared me to death, and the strange thing was that I didn't experience it as a problem with my vision. I really thought that part of the wall was missing...."

The doctor then picks up his microphone and says, "The patient suffered a scintillating and a negative scotoma."[139]

Shattering and fracturing the landscape, making the ordinary stream of visual imagery problematic and conditional, a migraine aura casts doubt on the basic nature and meaning of existence. The scotoma is an archaic, crude artifact, a gash that goes right from leaves on a tree or a child's face to the stuff of which the brain is made, churning up the entire fabric of light, cells, and synapses along the way. What this suggests is that auras originate within a very primitive psychophysiology (reptilian and older) and represent evolutionary as well as personal crises. Their motifs have to do with the roots of consciousness, the dawn of culture, and the birth of human identity.

II.
The Biology
of Migraine Auras

Aura Structure

An aura generally starts as a tiny defect and expands while traversing, dissipating where it previously existed. As its underlying garble spreads and captures more and more proprioceptive tracks, it is transformed by the feedback it generates. The expansion of a miniscule blinding dot into a full scotoma or mottle, the iteration of triangular or hexagonal artifacts, the development and transit of a complex shape across the field of vision, and the treacherously beautiful geometry of its permutations suggest uniform structural and geometrizing factors as well as a single source.

Likewise, a tactile aura—a prickling, itching, or numb spot—sprouts as a slight tingle at the fingertips, toetips, one fingertip or toetip, the tip of the tongue, etc., and spreads gradually across a hand, foot, or whole face without necessarily causing any other debility. Local and nonlocal, the sensation may then, while continuing to track at the site of origin (or not), spread to appendages, chest, or abdomen and/or travel toward and along the spine into the sacrum or skull.

A formication or paresthesia oscillates at the same frequency as a scotoma and, when it moves into the region of the head, like the scotoma it distorts speech and memory and undermines general cognitive function. When an aura descends into the stomach and intestines, it causes loss of bowel control and/or vomiting.

Regardless of the form of a migraine and its extant symptoms, the attack is expressed in a series of semi-congruent variances from "normal" functioning. Migraines are patterned discharges that jump across neural boundaries. They appear to be vested in a central cerebral episode or series of episodes—an elusive migraine germ—that, like the hard drive of a computer, affects components above it in particular ways. The fact that symptoms proceed along parallel trajectories in similar patterns, are dynamically equivalent, and can exchange with each other suggests their common source: "the same organization, expressed through homologous mechanisms at different levels."[1]

Lashley arrived at a similar conclusion years earlier, recognizing that a fundamental neurocognitive agency exerts omneity over ordinary syntaxes of perception and cognition. During hemianopia "filling in the blindspot and the completion of figures in scotomatous areas are not the results of habits of disregarding blind areas or of identifying parts of figures. The phenomena appear immediately with new blind areas. They must, then, represent some intrinsic organizing function of the cortex. The features completed are reduplicated patterns or very simple symmetric figures. The relation of this fact to the tendency to reduplication in fortification figures and other patterns of 'spontaneous' activity of the visual areas is suggestive of a common mechanism.

"Such phenomena can be made intelligible by the assumption that the integrative mechanism of the striate cortex tends to reproduce a pattern of excitation, aroused in one region, in any other region also if the latter is not dominated by different afferent patterns. Such a reduplication of patterns should result from the spreading of waves of excitation from points of initial stimulation, by analogy with the transmission of wave patterns on the surface of a liquid."[2]

While one person may experience an ocular aura; another, prickling in the appendages; another, dysphasia and alien visitors; another, some combination thereof—these are the same initial signal, outputs of the same mechanism. The underlying disposition is what a migraine aura *is,* not a scotoma or numbness. Each pathomechanism—whether auditory, visual, or tactile—is one manifestation.

Like a tidal wave, a migraine propagates as a whole, while its peculiar symptoms develop and spread idiosyncratically by locale and individual constitution. This would explain why migraine is sometimes a visual aura, sometimes a tinnitus, sometimes tingling.*

Sacks emphasizes this pandemic nature: "*Everything* comes and goes, nothing is settled, and if one could take a total thermogram, or scan, or inner photograph of the body, one would see vascular beds opening and closing, peristalsis accelerating or stopping, viscera squirming or tightening in spasms, secretions suddenly increasing or lessening—as if the nervous system was in a state of indecision."[3] He quotes an eminent novelist: "You keep pressing me to say that the attacks start with this symptom or that symptom, this phenomenon or that phenomenon, but this is not the way I experience them. It doesn't start with one symptom, it starts as a whole. You feel the whole thing, quite tiny at first, right from the start.... It's like glimpsing a point, a familiar point on the horizon, and gradually getting nearer, seeing it get larger and larger; or glimpsing your destination from far off, in a plane, having it get clearer and clearer as you descend through the clouds. The migraine *looms,* but it's just a change of scale—everything is always there from the start."[4] (Ellipses and italics his.)

Migraines represent an extremely complex, multiform, and profound *potential* field of visions, distortions, apparitions, seizures, and disorientations, out of which only a few are actually *seen or felt* in any one episode. Others may be intimated and latent, which is another reason why global unease accompanies the phenomenon and also why an acute headache often follows. The actual neurological shift is far denser than initially comprehended.

---

*A point easily missed: the headache and vomiting are not *aura* symptoms, as the pathomechanisms of the various forms of aura are different from those underlying sheer pain.

History of Medical Research*

From the birth of medical science, migraines and their auras have been investigated by a number of scientists and physicians. Before it was understood that they were relatively benign, some researchers thought that they might originate in acute brain pathology. Thus mid-nineteenth- to mid-twentieth-century physicians took them quite seriously and sought their cause in a malady with differential expressions.

To begin with what seems most empirically obvious, migraines occur in the brain and central nervous system and encompass consecutive cycles of neural and cerebral excitation and inhibition. Initial aura arousal, including phosphenes, colorings, and abstract shapes, actually replicates quite closely what happens when the cortex is excited directly: artificial electrical stimulation of the primary visual cortex or its surrounding association areas results in flickering, dancing patterns and sparks similar to those of migraine auras.

Changes in consciousness and perception, including disorien-

---

*I believe that I have fairly summarized past and current medical literature on migraine auras in this section, but I should confess that an old college classmate who is a neurologist looked at my text, perhaps cursorily, and emailed me back that "modern-day molecular biology is poorly addressed with a lot of antiquated theories of migraine pathogenesis." I am not sure that he doesn't have an axe to grind here, because he *really* didn't like my discussion of alternative modalities in the next section. Regardless of his critique, I cannot draw a firm line anywhere, from the nineteenth into the twenty-first century, between scientific migraine myths and scientific migraine facts. The line he might draw would lead to a more unilinear, moleculocentric, genetically deterministic etiology than the evidence suggests. When I asked him for references to better theories, he declined to be more specific than the above, which suggests to me politics more than biology. I will leave any additional judgments to my readers.

tation and unconscious spells, might be associated with some sort of blockage, vasoconstriction, or aggravation of the brainstem and reticular formation.

Sacks categorizes a migraine as an autonomous disturbance of unknown origin in the deep brain, probably the brainstem, with an abnormal firing of neurons that discharges upward into the visual cortex, stirring intrinsic activity in the visual field like an extremely vivid, non-narrative waking dream, and, from there, into the association areas where it overstimulates other cortical neurons—in other words, a deviant event in the brainstem nuclei, possibly from a chemical source, gathering upward momentum with increasing feedback.[5] He summarizes these dynamics:

"[T]here must be massive, slow potentials emanating from the brainstem, and projected from this both 'upstream' and 'downstream' in the nervous system," distracting ultimately the visual and other zones of the cortex, the periaqueductal grey matter, and raphé nuclei, and even the spinal cord, also constricting cortical microcirculation, and of course initiating visual and other "aural" effects.[6] Hyperactivity of noradrenergic and serotonergic systems in the brainstem, once aroused, could give rise to some of the throbbing and hallucinations.

Migraine can thus be represented as a signal from deep under the surface that gets translated into discrete patternings as it encounters structures along the way and is received and processed by a neurocerebral apparatus. The scotoma is fashioned by configurations of the visual cortex and its optic recognition nuclei, as well as organizational predilections of the greater brain in response to intrinsic stimulation, and synergistic feedback loops that expand, diversify, and transform the emerging hallucination, becoming phases which pass across the field of vision as the vanguard of an excitation/inhibition wave. Electrical activity in the cortex is stimulated and then dampened, e.g. flashing lights are followed by a blacking out of vision.

Causes for migraines proposed over more than a century address hormonal imbalance, neurological discharges, vascular reactivity, microcirculation, oxygen deficiency in sensitive regions of the brain, and compromises of blood-flow to the brain. Migraines are cumulatively defined as microcirculatory disorders, summarized in vasoconstriction and sympathetic hyperactivity, leading to diminishment of cerebral oxygen and overall obstructed flow of blood and nourishment through the nervous system. Etiological interrelationships of these factors remain poorly understood, and some scientists provide completely other rationales. Here is the range of about a century and a half of explanations that I find in books, articles, and online (with repetition and overlap to allow for nomenclature of slightly differing interpretations plus limitations of my own anatomical knowledge):[7]

- a build-up of blood in the arteries of the brain;
- a local obstruction to cerebral arterial flow;
- congestion of the venous system of the brain;
- a broad vasomotor dysfunction or nerve storms, e.g. electrical disturbances of the brain itself;
- abnormalities of platelet function;
- arterial spasm from sympathetic stimulation;
- a spreading cortical depression;
- a unilateral failure of the vasomotor nerves of the carotid artery, leading the artery to relax, hence a diminishing supply of blood to the brain with the vessels in the brain contracting—a cycle instigated by excited action of the sympathetic nervous system and relieved by dilation of the same vessels after the sympathetic action has exhausted itself;
- oxygen deficiency in critical regions of the brain, requiring compensatory vascular dilation;
- cerebral vasoconstriction/vasodilation with local anemia— modern researchers are more or less divided between those who

deem that the vasospasm is secondary and those who think it is central and arises from a mutation in a polymorphic gene that governs a vasoconstrictor, endothelin type A receptor (ETA-231A/G);

• overall destabilization of the nervous system such that when unsettled neural activity reaches a certain point, neurohormonal homeostasis is disturbed, leading to a train of paroxysmal effects, no one of which could incite a migraine—much as a strategic scratch on a piece of unannealed glass causes the entire sheet to crumble;

• aggravation of peripheral nerves among visceral, muscular, or cutaneous components;

• an abnormal sensitivity to sensory inputs in general (this is not an originating cause but a co-factor);

• the descent of an irritation from higher cognitive and emotional centers;

• extreme histamine sensitivity;

• an increase in the level of acetylcholine in the spinal fluid;

• a sudden decline in the ratio of circulating serotonin leading, by a rebound mechanism, to a bloating of extracranial vessels;

• lesions discharging out of the optic thalamus, corresponding closely enough to epilepsy to be a form of epilepsy;

• cerebral lesions;

• changes in brain chemistry, including abruptly peaking levels of neurotransmitters like serotonin or dopamine;

• a relationship among cortical depression, neurotransmitters, genetic codes, and the dura mater such that various enzymes are released and breach the blood-brain barrier;[8]

• bacterial infection by *Helicobacter pylori* (advanced as the cause of about forty percent of all migraines by A. Gasbarrini and associates in a 1998 issue of *Hepatogastroenterology*);[9]

• an abnormal opening (the patent foramen ovale or PFO) between the heart's upper chambers after fetal development, allowing circulating blood to by-pass the lungs (which are not used for breathing in the womb): when this one-way shunt remains open in some people, it releases air bubbles, dissolved chemicals, debris, and sometimes clots to the head, causing abnormal neurological activity, auras, etc.[10]

All of these theories depict physicochemical aspects of migraines, be they causes or effects, originating factors or concomitances. As in the Sufi fable of blind men interrogating an elephant with their hands such that each comes away with a different description of the animal from landing upon a unique part of the anatomy (ears, trunk, tail, feet, etc.), so researchers of migraines who do not take into account the holistic nature of the condition generally valorize some partial aspect of its physiology and etiology, missing others.

Theories that attempt to define diffuse multifocal phenomena in terms of singular, linear physiological and/or biochemical elements tend to suffer from misplaced concreteness and lead to errors and unsuccessful treatments. For instance (as noted elsewhere), there is no paradigm of migraine that can be confirmed by blood tests, imaging devices, or other research; and no identifiable biochemical activity, by its increase or diminution, is a confident antecedent of migraines or auras.

Where would one hunt for the format of a migraine? Historically scientists have looked for microanatomical constraints that could explain or represent auras and their structuring on the assumption that there must be concrete elements in the brain and eye—cerebral, optic, and general neural structures and hard-wired pathways—shaping such hallucinations, even as there are geologies lodged within the contours of weather systems.

The nineteenth-century author J. F. W. Herschel, while tracking his own "fortification, with salient and re-entering angles, bastions, and ravelins," wondered whether he was staring at the morphology of the eye and concluded that the motifs could *not* have been caused by any "possible regularity of structure in the retina or optic nerve."[11] Anticipating snowflake-like and branchlike self-similar patterns that would become familiar to mathematicians nearly a century later in Mandelbrot and Julia sets, he proposed that aura imagery must be generated "from an impersonal and unconscious part of the mind— an elemental 'geometrizing' part of the [higher] brain ... 'distinct from that of our own personality ... a kaleidoscopic power in the sensorium to form regular patterns by the symmetrical combination of casual elements.'"[12]

In 1904 Gowers interpreted the fortification spectra as an imprint of colliding neural phenomena even as banks of clouds represent intersections of humidity and pressure in fronts: "[I]ts well-known curved character ... seems to be due to some opposing forces in the process, by which the discharge in a straight line cannot proceed beyond a short distance and is then compelled to give place to one at right angles to it."[13]

K. S. Lashley, having access to more advanced biology in the early 1940s, speculated that "although nothing is known of the actual nervous activity during the migraine, the picture suggests that the propagated disturbance is so intense as to be independent of the afferent supply of the cortex and that the pattern represents the type of organization into which the cortical activity falls as a result of inherent properties of the architectonic structure."[14]

The 1960s confirmed the existence of "architectonic structures which might be organizing the excitation ... a variety of 'feature detectors' within the visual cortex ... organized into small 'columns' ... 'straight-lined angular forms' ..." with fortifications and ravelins as described by Herschel. This "suggests that the neurons of the cortex being activated either have such orientations themselves (if there is a literal correspondence between cortical patterns and hallucinatory patterns), or are sensitive to different orientations."[15]

He concludes that the advancing excitation wave associated with a scotoma activates preexisting pools of columns as it crosses them, one after another, throwing them into activity, causing bars of light to arrange themselves in shining simulation, column by column. "In this way, the migraine fortification is an excellent natural experiment: the advancing waves of disturbance draw continuous traces across the cortex and in less than half an hour reveal part of the secret of its neuronal organization."[16]

In the period after World War I, German researcher Johann Hoffman conducted one of the earliest scientific experiments with migraine auras, using a simple matching test to arrive at a flicker rate for scotomata at 10 Hz, which turns out also to be the range of alpha rhythms in an electroencephalogram (EEG). Later EEG readings showed "abnormalities of many kinds in connection with migraine—generalized slow-wave disrhythmias, convulsive patterns, focal abnormalities," etc., during the passage of scotomata.[17] In the early 1970s, Danish microcirculation measurements of cerebral blood flow with radioactive tracers in animals (the morality of which we will let pass for the moment) showed a spreading depression wave of reduced blood flow in the cerebral cortex at the same rate as scotomata (of course without reference to any hallucinations themselves, since animals do not report).

In 1985 intracarotid injection of xenon into patients with classic migraine disclosed that "regional cerebral blood flow was reduced during the aura, beginning in the occipital area and gradually spreading anteriorly over the entire hemisphere. The reduction did not heed vascular territories, but instead seemed to respect architectonic zones such as the central sulcus and sylvan fissure."[18] Interestingly, the researchers could not find equivalent decreases in patients with common (auraless) migraines, nor could they demonstrate compensatory regions of later *increased* flow, so the application of the study to migraine is unclear.

In the early 1990s microencephalographic measurements of the human brain's neuromagnetic fields through the skull confirmed a wave "with excited spikes at its advancing rim and depressed slow waves in their wake, mov[ing] across the visual cortex at 2 to 3 millimeters per minute during visual migraine auras."[19] While corroborating a physical basis for scotomata, this may well say more about the effects of a migraine than its causes: one expects electrical outbursts from a storm, but they are not the storm's source.

Recent technology has allowed the consideration of brain lesions as explanations for auras and aura-like phenomena. The 1998 Israeli investigation of reversal-of-vision metamorphopsia mentioned on p. 66, though not a study of migraine *per se*, speculates "that a separate mechanism of visual orientation might exist in each cerebral hemisphere and that occipital and parietal lesions that spare the optic radiations may account for the oblique [less than 180 degrees] and complete RVM." They conclude that "failure to perceive space in an allocentric coordinate frame, particularly in the coronal roll plane, is potentially the critical event underlying RVM."[20]

In 2003, MRI scans revealed white-matter lesions in 12–47 percent of young persons experiencing regular migraines as opposed to 2–14 percent in control groups.[21] The pathological relationship of these to actual headaches or auras, if any, is unknown, as they may indicate comorbidities, chance findings, or concurrent ailments.*

---

*These relate to metalloproteinase models of migraine-transit leakage through the blood-brain barrier: "Application of matrix metalloproteinase models to migraine helps explain the ability of medications to cross the blood-brain barrier during a migraine episode, as well as describe possible ischaemia with repeated migraine (e.g. white matter abnormalities ...)."[22]

Still unexplained by any experiments or studies are the coincidence or semi-coincidence of headaches with auras; the greater sensitivity of the visual cortex than the cutaneous-kinesthetic or auditory cortices; the long and subtle migrainous prodrome giving rise to hallucinations; auras' emotional components, including mania, elation, anxiety, and the like; and the manifold complexity of an aura with its permuting fields and self-replication by fractal diffusion as compared to other symptoms elicited by stimulation of the visual cortex, vascular constriction, or variable neurotransmitter levels in the brain. That is, migraine auras deliver a lot more psychoneural punch and intricate design than straightforward depression waves, vascular constrictions, and related biochemical loci would seem to account for. Additionally, there are the chameleon and self-transforming qualities of the aura (such to appear in myriad guises and motifs); the arousal of second and sometimes subsequent scotomata after the first has passed, in contradiction to a simple two-stage cycle of constriction and dilation marking onset and decline; the unusual flicker-rate of the scotoma; and the way that one migraine equivalent exchanges psychosomatic identity with another and morphs into it. Sacks concludes: "It is impossible to explain the varying levels and transformations of migraine in terms of fixed neural mechanisms."[23]

An even more complex system of organization (or disorganization) would be necessary to derive multiple lattices, mosaics, spiraling and conical shapes, the shrinking and expansion of objects, Turkish carpets, and radiolaria patterns—not only how such patterns could occur but how they mutate and serialize. Hallucinations like the rearrangement of time and space, the inability to recognize familiar objects (agnosia)—let alone miniature oxen and whole nonexistent guests—do not correspond to anything generated by primary stimulation of the visual cortex or vasoconstriction and are even beyond the kinds of hallucinations caused by stimulation of the secondary, tertiary, and peripheral zones of the cortex. Sacks guesses that advanced functions beginning in secondary fields generate complex hallucinations and phantoms, culminating in a plethora of successive confused states incorporating one another until the excitation passes.[24]

While auras emerge from neuron clusters in the hypothalamus and below, i.e., "from some abnormal neural activity or reactivity deep in the brainstem ..." likely involving tonic changes of brainstem excitation and inhibition and the alignment of the autonomic nervous system,[25] their "iconography" is expressed in "functional schematization *above* anatomically fixed cytoarchitectonic patterns."[26] As complication flows upward, it enlists the broader electrochemistry of the nervous system, encompassing cortical excitation and spreading into cerebral and psychosomatic mechanisms.

Taking such factors and the sum of neurological research into account, Sacks arrives at a picture of "a form of centrencephalic seizure, the activity of which is projected rostrally upon the cerebral hemispheres, and peripherally via the ramifications of the autonomic nervous system.... [T]he cortex is subjected to an ascending bombardment in the course of a migraine aura, to which it responds with secondary activities of its own."[27] These include phosphenes, scotomata, and other diffuse effects. Thereupon the peripheral autonomic plexuses are susceptible to a "descending barrage to which they respond with secondary, multifocal activities of their own."[28]

As a feedback cycle is spawned, other systems get pulled into it, including "convergence in the spinal nerve of afferent fibres from the upper three cervical nerves with the descending tract of the trigeminal nerve, [meaning] that pain can be referred from the neck to the temples and back again."[29] As trigeminal impulses and their effects amplify extracranial blood flow and reinforce one another, they elicit more sensation and vasodilation, broadening the overall symptomology.

A contemporary (2004) neurologist in Madrid offers a variant of this model based on subsequent research. He submits that pathogenesis of the later (upper cerebral) phases of classic migraines (aura followed by headache) is a multilevel cortical episode, leading to activation of sensitive structures in the cerebral/neural nexus (trigeminovascular pathways) and causing chemical changes that have, at minimum, secondary and tertiary consequences of Rube Goldberg proportions. Ignition is seminal and deep-seated, enlisting genetic codes and molecular/enzymatic mechanisms:

"[E]vidence that cortical spreading depression is the underlying pathomechanism of migraine aura has increased.... It has been debated how a primarily cortical phenomenon (aural phase) may activate trigeminal fibres (headache phase). Recent data have demonstrated a link between cortical events and activation of the pain-sensitive structures of the dura mater. The initial cortical hyperfusion in cortical spreading depression is partly mediated by the release of trigeminal and parasympathetic neurotransmitters from perivascular nerve fibres, whereas delayed meningeal blood flow increase is mediated by trigeminal-parasympathetic brainstem connection. With regard to molecular mechanisms, cortical spreading depression unregulates a variety of genes coding for COX-2, TNF-alpha, IL-1beta, galanin or metalloproteinases. The activation of metalloproteinases leads to leakage of the blood-brain barrier, allowing potassium, nitric oxide, adenosine, and other products released by cortical spreading depression to reach and sensitize the dural perivascular trigeminal afferents. In familial hemiplegic migraine, new mutations have been described in chromosome 1q23, leading to a haploinsufficiency of the sodium/potassium pump, producing an increase in intracellular calcium...."[30]

Instead of (or in addition to) single chemiconeural triggers and complex hierarchies, we recognize nowadays that migraines represent dynamic disequilibrium of the nervous system as a whole, and their microstates are more likely triggered by a convergence of co-factors than any one intrinsic thing (for instance, a bad night's sleep combined with chronic stress plus a sudden unpleasant odor during a period of vascular, enzymatic, and/or neural susceptibility). It is possible that a discharge from the brainstem is merely one stage in a sequence initiated circumstantially by menstruation; an allergy; a change in humidity, temperature, or altitude; a full moon, whatever.

If migraines express necessary activity in the homeostasis of an organism, then any particular individual initiating mechanism may be random; if it is suppressed, the aura will still find another outlet for signification. As adaptive, coping mechanisms with multiple channels of expression, migraines are going to discharge their components via one pathway or another. As chaotic, decoherent, nonlinear phenomena, they have the power to override the inactivation of any one element of their charge. When the cumulative surge of a dimensionless depression in the nervous system builds up to critical mass, it explodes like a thunderstorm with lightning and hail, and sweeps all parts into revelation, whether particular organs are proximally activated or not.

Migraines begin everywhere and nowhere, are developmentally and somatically collateral, and encompass anything in the organism, though not everything every time. Artifacts of the deeper brain in their atavistic arousal and core excitation, they are epiphenomena of the higher cerebral naves in their quasi-semantic expression and abstract, imaginal displays. Like many other neurological and psychedelic discharges, auras produce a phenomenology that dramatically exceeds anything that is detected physiologically or biochemically in the brain. Though they certainly have discernible sources and leave trails, they audaciously generate an entire cinema and their own mode of consciousness above them.

Other Migrainous and Migrainoid Phenomena

*Migraine Equivalents, Migraine-like States, and Migrainoid
Phenomena*

Even as migraines are polymorphous in their symptomology and
expression, they are also one of a fundamental class of events in
which the body-mind responds to a stimulus with cyclical paroxysmal and/or hallucinatory effects. Individual migraine manifestations thus characterize broader or more fundamental patterns.

Sacks uses the term "migraine equivalent" for symptoms that are
migrainous in character but lack a headache—homologous components organized in different sequences. Standard migraine equivalents include migraine auras (of course); spasms of abdominal pain
and vomiting; fevers; disruptions of kinesthesia; discrete fugues of
drowsiness, nausea, and vomiting; psychological disorientation;
transitory spates of dizziness or local numbness; and otherwise inexplicable pains.[31]

An astonishingly diverse range of additional pleasurable, semi-
pleasurable, unpleasurable, and uncategorizable events likewise per-
mutes along a "migraine" spectrum. Loosely following Sacks, I will
call most of these "migrainoid" rather than "migrainous." Sacks
distinguishes "migrainoid episodes" from migraines or migraine
equivalents (though the distinction is fluid and arbitrary). The former—some more closely than others—resemble migraines in
aspects of their etiology, structure, and symptoms, but they also
diverge in key characteristics. The world of migrainoid phenomena
ranges from "dramatic and sudden collapse[s] to protracted autonomic reactions with haziness, but not loss, of consciousness."[32]
Among its more conspicuous events are vagal attacks; faints; pro-
tective fright reactions; swoons (from being overcome with emotion); vertigos; narcolepsies; cataplexies (losses of muscle power);
hysterical, depressive, and catatonic stupors; neuralgias; and motion

sickness. More serious brain pathologies and seizures like epilepsy and Parkinson's symptoms are also migrainoid by way of their acute and passive neural qualities.[33]

In the instance of the woman mentioned by Gowers on page 33, migraines were replaced by epileptic attacks, suggesting a core equivalence on some neurological or psychoneural level: "The patient, after suffering from migraine for many years, became the subject of epilepsy, the migraine ceasing when the epileptic fits commenced. This transition is not infrequent, and that it was really such is shown by the unusual fact that the visual prodroma of the attacks of migraine became the warning of the epileptic fits, in more rapid evolution."[34]

An unspecific complex of loosely allied conditions is probably operating through the neuroendocrine system; for instance, studies have shown that migraines run in higher percentages in families which also have allergies, muscle-contraction headaches, arthritis, hypertension, attention deficit, and other cerebrovascular and nervous or psychological disorders.

To a mixed migrainoid-migrainous spectrum, I will add involuntary tics and partially involuntary reactions like shivering, vomiting (e.g. from thought of something disgusting), sneezes, laughter (from tickling), laughter (from something funny), hiccoughs, and even the stimulation and tumescence of sexual organs.

A broader migrainoid range would include drunkenness; hangovers; hay fever; drug reactions (when causing restlessness, belching, cold sweats, and/or drowsiness); visceral dilations following injuries; night sweats and salivations; sleep paralysis and other hypnogogic and dreamlike phenomena; restless legs; migraine-equivalent, partially psychosomatic illnesses (asthma, peptic ulcers, insomnia); and the parallel realm of somatopsychic diseases like panics, chronic depression, obsessive compulsions, hysterias, neuroses, and phobias.[35] Except for the pain and nausea that some experience, migraines are blithe and emotionally neutral by comparison with anxiety, and proprioceptively superficial by comparison with sex (discharging more like a tic or Tourette's syndrome).

Awareness and responsiveness enable a recipient either to enhance or constrict many migrainoid experiences in different ways to affect their quality, depth, and quantum of discharge. Typically humans amplify and fixate erotic fantasies to increase excitement; yet they also, consciously or unconsciously, quash the same expressions. The relation between active thought and spasmodic release is a subtle one, playing quite different roles in laughter, seduction, sneezing, and migraines. Our mind-body feedback accommodates varying degrees of receptivity to and inhibition of stimulation, which dramatically impact their expressions: a suppressed sneeze (or giggle) is different from a spontaneous one; likewise, a reflected-upon phobia is less rigid than an unexamined one. Yet these acts all encompass migrainoid gradients and discharge patterns. Though most of them are not conventionally libidinal—have not picked up significant characterological force from instinctual drives or wish-fulfillment fantasies—that does not mean that they do not embody protolibidinal aspects that generally attend arousal and orgasm. I surmise that migraine auras are somewhat orgasmic and semeiological, but not particularly Oedipal or erotic.

Despite the variations and differences, what enables us to categorize migrainous/migrainoid expression is the identification of a range of somatic and psychosomatic phenomena incurring spasms, inhibitions, and discharges. Migraine auras belong to a class of body-mind spasms that comprise cycles (brief or protracted) of arousal, augmentation, and discharge, some more migrainoid than others. As we shall see in the next section, their migrainoid aspect conceivably marks their position on an evolutionary ladder from tropismic arousal to full consciousness. The more migrainoid acts are usually more primitive, but these stages are not purely hierarchical and can represent other adaptive factors and epigenetic innovations including fetal and paedomorphic mutations.

Motion Sickness

The kinship between migraines and motion sickness tells us much about both maladies—they are paroxysms resulting in temporarily durable (as opposed to fleeting) psychophysiological bouts of nausea and dizziness ("scotoma"), each comprising a distortion of balance, each irreconcilable. The aggravations are different but related (more nausea and vertigo in motion sickness; more pain and/or explicit hallucinations in migraines; disorientation, intestinal upset, cataplexy, and enfeeblement in both). Parenthetically, a number of researchers have commented on the complement of people (close to half, in fact) who suffered motion sickness, either in childhood or continuing into adult life, and then migraines, often beginning after episodes of motion sickness ended (usually during adolescence)—a replacement cycle. Apparently migraines and motion sickness share cerebral roots and arousal pathways. Sufferers of seasickness, carsickness, spacesickness, etc., are hypersensitive to changes in orientation, movement, and locations of objects in relation to one another (and self), while those experiencing auras are susceptible to various sorts of anomalies, blurs, and deviations in the visual field.

Motion sickness was once presumed to be a mostly physical ailment from combined effects of shifting cerebrospinal fluid, imbalance in the cochlear flow in the inner ear, microgravitational influences on organs, vestibular overload, and uncoordinated head-eye movements. Because fluid in the inner ear regulates our sense of balance, variations in its biophysics were thought to be a primary cause of the dizziness, nausea, and disorientation associated with motion sickness.

Throughout the last decades of the twentieth century, NASA (the

American space agency), which has vested interest in the ailment because of astronauts' proneness to it during liftoff and in the weightless environment of space, conducted experiments with men and women in floating dizziness-inducing capsules and other simulated environments. It turned out that motion sickness is instigated at least as much in the brain and mind as it is in the inner ear.[36] When the mind predicts that objects should fall into a particular conformation and they do not, e.g. when the landscape does not match a person's expectation of his or her surroundings—and especially when one thinks he or she is about to go in one direction and the thrust of a vehicle (or gravityless space) takes them in another—in some people a secondary, far more potent and bottomless disorientation arises, a collapse induced more by its own dissonant feedback than a mere flub in a kinesthetic message. Much as the body tries to adjust to the real situation, an auxiliary fixation continues to spread such that disorientation pathologizes into a miasm. A predictable sequence of effects follows: loss of mental and physical clarity, convulsions, nausea, vertigo, vitiation.

Like scotomata, motion sickness strikes at the core of being. As afflicted aquanauts and astronauts across epochs will attest, few malignancies—even ones far more severe and deep-seated—are so uncomfortable and decimating. Most would rather die than go on suffering such nausea and dizziness indefinitely, despite the fact that motion sickness is *not* a serious disease.

Migraines and motion sickness share a precipice quality; before an elusive tipping point at which dissonant elements get their claws in, one can reverse course and flee the gathering maelstrom unscathed (symptoms dissipate quickly). Once the initial, often intangible throes have been registered, a threshold has been passed and there is no way out of the spasm except through its other end—and no way extrinsically to deconstruct or antidote the event. After onset, the symptoms—disorientating nausea in motion sickness and hallucinations and blindness from a scotoma—become self-inducing. Attempts to abort them, even drugs that are somewhat successful, imbue vestigial complications that drag out the deficits.

Each ailment is a one-way street, a roller-coaster that cannot be halted. Once a person crosses a brink into a new neural universe, his body loses some of its sense of reality. Each condition expands into a fog of such saturation that it seems as though it will never dissipate—and nothing else is of any importance while it is happening. Yet migraine auras and motion-induced nauseas always conclude peacefully, even if, while elapsing, they are torturous—and however severe and debilitating, however timeless and incapacitating, they abate without transferring any lasting pathology. They leave pretty much a clean slate.

Both conditions also impart profound and enigmatic emotional qualities; both have an ancient plan that is the same every time, a ritual to enact, a narrative structure with its own beginning, middle, and end: "Being lost in the Underworld, I recover on the other side of my pilgrimage and find myself possessed of new energy and power." This primal myth inspired tales like *Batman* and *Superman*—a poisoning or catastrophe leads to ego death followed by rebirth in heroic form. The migrainous body may be the antithesis of the superhero body (weakened rather than enhanced) but, in being opposite, it is the cauldron in which the latter is forged.

Migraines and motion sickness are waking, palpable, tactile dreams (or nightmares); brief psychotic vigils and transits through a shadow realm in which opportunities for psychosomatic death and metamorphosis are conferred.

Trances

While auras are temporary mottles and holes in visual fabrics, dreams are wholesale shifts of virtual reality—tuning fork, coverlet, and curtain. Fully convincing hallucinations that are as cohesive as a movie or exotic excursion, they are like entire afternoons in lives.

Scotomata are not dreamlike in either their phenomenology or capacity to induce beguiling trances, so they fall at one end of a gradient that has them at the pure "migraine" pole, and dreams at the opposite, "hypnotic trance" pole. In the middle (along with motion sickness) are all sorts of closed- and open-eye migrainoid phantasms—hypnogogic tremors, mirages, sleepwalking, and comas, as well as highly paradoxical and confusing thoughts mixed with images, fleeting memories and misremembered things, and brief paroxysms and starts that are instantly forgotten. We tend to ignore such basal artifacts because what interests us is the evolved scenery of the upper cortical levels of consciousness, i.e., what we call life.

Hollywood hypnotists—as well as many professional therapists—put their subjects in trances by swinging an object like a pocket watch in front of them in pendulum fashion, evoking a fixation. Counting backwards is another hypnosis-inducing technique that has migrainous aspects, e.g. acalculia. Hypnotists may give their thralls subliminal instructions that are then carried out even after they are "awake" and out of a hypnotized state. The subjects respond to these commands as if motivated by events in the world.

Certain schools of philosophers and Buddhist meditators consider reality itself an especially vivid hypnotic trance—one of a variety of illusory vibrations into which sentient beings tune across a multidimensional universe. Along this spectrum of conditional realities exist incalculable discrete frequencies, each representing its own illusorily "real" world, yet each in effect a "migrainoid" phantasm. Realities are made solely of stuff like atoms that are mostly space and potential. We inhabit these by signals between our cells: worlds exist solely in brains.

Reality-testing and lucid dreaming (awaking within dream to know one is dreaming) can be viewed as trans-migrainoid states through which one emerges—instructed—out of one level of trance into another, ostensibly higher one. This speaks also to the awakening of the animal kingdom on Earth into self-awareness and knowledge—the evolution of consciousness, an epochal migrainoid legacy.

Telepathy

Psychedelic trips and various other hallucinogenic and parapsychological states have migrainoid attributes. People ingesting substances to arouse a primitive substrate, either recreationally or as part of a spiritual practice, experience altered modes of consciousness and meta-perceptual realities. These visions, ranging from ecstatic epiphanies to psychotomimetic stupors, generate eerie landscapes, autonomous spirits, and borderline personages—messengers from unknown parts of ourselves or perhaps the paraphysical universe.

Assorted telepathies, acts of remote viewing, and incipient telekineses (if they ever mature into real skills in us) could be "explained" futuristically as higher-order migrainoid functions. Surplus cerebral artifacts and diseases like Tourette's syndrome and epilepsy might point to untapped neural capacities, even as migraines themselves are probably remnants of archaeological phases. Aptitudes that are currently in ascendance, after all, developed from little more than arousal and inhibition waves in simple bionts. If scotomata are leftover shards of primitive consciousness, then they and some other migrainoid states might be forerunners of advanced modes of cognition (see p. 139).

Alien Abductions

Accounts from reputed UFO abductees have a distinct migrainoid ring to them: inexplicable lights, missing time, humanoid or animal-headed creatures—though these matters of course raise other ontological issues. Attribution of migrainoid qualities addresses the neural component of such "close encounters"; it is not to say that there are no alien abductions (whether or not there are is not the province of this book), merely to note that these episodes share elements with fugues that originate in the brainstem. Encounters with aliens—fairies, ghosts, angels, and disembodied spirits among them—might be actual metaphysical meetings and yet evoke migrainoid vestiges, falsifying the entities. This suggests the humorous maxim that, just because one is paranoid doesn't mean someone isn't out to get him.

Internal Pictures

Back toward the migrainous end of the migraine/trance gradient are conscious streams of images that occasionally run past closed-eye vision at such a speed that they seem still frames illumined on a movie reel passing through a projector in the ocular cortex—faces and landscapes and anomalous objects and views, many of them diagonally oriented or peephole-like, transiting at an astonishing ten to fifteen per second, each of them fully formed and lucid, no one of them thematically related to the one before or after it (or to anything, for that matter), each one gone and replaced in a microsecond. These spontaneous, self-made movies are dreamlike, high-speed cousins to auras—the closest approximation to a fusion of dream and migraine imagery.

In an aura, reality usually seems to have slowed down; in a conveyor belt of images, it has clearly speeded up—but emotionally somehow *both are the same thing*. In fact, both are high-speed flickers—one pictorial and tame, the other (scotomata) abstract and acute.

In a migrainous vision from childhood, probably a hypnogogic event of some kind, a sixteenth-century Italian physician remembered seeing "images of castles, of houses, of animals, of horses with rider, of plants and trees, of musical instruments, and of theaters; there were images of men of divers costumes and varied dress; images of flute-players, even with their pipes as it were, ready to play, but no voice or sound was heard. Besides these visions, I beheld soldiers, swarming peoples, fields, and shapes like unto bodies which even to this day I recall with aversion. There were groves, forests, and other phantoms which I no longer remember; at times I could see a veritable chaos of innumerable objects rushing dizzily along *en masse,* without confusion among themselves, yet with terrific speed. These images were, moreover, transparent, but not to such a degree that it was as if they were not, nor yet so dense as to be impenetrable to the eyes; rather the tiny rings were opaque and the spaces transparent.... Even flowers of many a variety, and four-footed creatures appeared in my vision....

"I was not a little delighted ... and gazed so raptly upon these marvels, that my aunt on one occasion questioned me whether I saw aught....

"Following the period of visions, I scarcely ever, until nearly daybreak, had any warmth from my knees down."[37]

I experienced a similarly hypnogogic vision during grade-school years whereby, while lying in bed waiting to fall asleep, I felt my fingers, toes, and sometimes also my limbs becoming paradoxically both denser and spongier, and changing distance so that they were very close and then suddenly very far away. The variations in distance correlated with a sensation of relative thickness. When my appendages were close, they were huge, and my mind seemed as much in the fabric of my fattened fingers or feet as it was in my head or any more familiar psychophysical place. It was as though I could instantaneously transport my ego down my body through the porosity of its parts, its passage making them bulbous and gigantic. Organs of the same quality of sensation became tactilely and anatomically the same organ or one discontinuous organ.

At times my feet seemed to accordion so close to my upper torso that they became part of the same dense mush as my fingers such that there was no distinction between them. I felt not even so much that my organs had moved to inappropriate places as that the benchmark of reality had changed and, instead of having fingers and toes, or even separate organs and shapes, I existed as areas of relative density and I located myself by their geography in my body—"my" position in relation to them—and I experienced my scale solely by this sponginess and its relative orientation. The hallucination replaced a more usual limbed-torso Vitruvian map.

In a correlative hallucination, often a sequel to the above, I would see a city or village at a very great distance and then instantaneously be inside it; then I would return to faraway. It was as though I were hovering over the village, and suddenly in it, and just as suddenly seeing it from above the whole Earth, then walking on one of its streets. These vistas occurred in such rapid and instantaneous succession that they did not seem segues in a movie but more like complete transformations of the nature of body and mind such that, with each propulsion, I was in a fresh relationship to the village and this was also a new aspect of my body.

None of these episodes had any association with pain or an aura, and they were pleasurable enough that I tried to elicit them throughout childhood and found I could play with and direct them like a cinematographer. Unlike the lock of an aura, I could snap out of their trance in an instant by stirring myself—though it might be difficult to get back in. If my exit was brief, I might slide back in by remembering the sensation or suggesting it to myself. After a few minutes, though, it was impossible to reenter until the state arose again, perhaps months later.

These trances occurred periodically from my earliest memories, always at night in bed, and then concluded, close to adolescence, at least thirty-six years before I experienced my first migraine aura; yet I feel they implicitly foreshadowed it.

Meditation Experiences

The arising of visual phenomena during states of deep concentration is well-documented within various Eastern meditative traditions. Some of these experiences were described by Swami Sivananda who, before becoming one of the twentieth century's most influential yogis, was an established medical doctor. He explained that while developing one's concentration, "when the eyes are closed, different coloured lights, white, yellow, red, smoky, blue, green, mixed lights, flashes like lightning, like fire, burning charcoal, fire-flies, moon, sun, stars" may appear.[38] These are said to be "elemental lights," each element—earth, water, fire, air—having its respective color. Their appearance is regarded not as anything special, but merely the result of progress in one's ability to concentrate. And so the would-be meditator is advised to not be distracted by them, but instead to "shun them" while trying to "dive deep into their source," which is nothing more than the mind itself.

Within the Tibetan Buddhist traditions the experiences that occur during meditation are generally described as falling into one of two basic types: "distractions" or "sidetracks" and "signs of progress." The various random visual occurrences that may appear during the fundamental practice of concentration known as "shamatha" or "calm abiding" are said to be the result of the movement of the "karmic wind." The breath and the mind are seen to be linked and thus the various visual phenomena are regarded as little more than the result of an undisciplined mind and, as one achieves ever deeper states of calm, these phenomena diminish. Later, in the still quite secret practices of the Dzogchen tradition known as *tögal,* diverse stable visions unfold as signs of progress through the final stages before complete enlightenment. Through a combination of body posture and specific eye gazes the "vajra chain of awareness" appears in any of numerous forms such as knots tied in a strand of a horse's tail, a string of pearls, fish eggs, etc. As one's practice evolves, these stabilize and other more elaborate manifestations unfold such as radiant lattices of light, spear-points, a thousand-petalled lotus flower etc. Over time one's awareness is maintained unbroken in ever longer stretches, at which point circles or spheres may appear, sometimes similar to rhinoceros-skin shields. These begin to grow in size until the light pervades everywhere one looks.[39]

Perhaps the lights, shapes, mandalas, etc., that appear during meditation are due to neural alterations caused by practice and may be similar to the patterns or disruptions which cause migraine auras. In Tibetan medicine the concept of "lung," which is most often translated as "wind," would be used to diagnose, explain, and treat such conditions as migraines and auras, these being little more than imbalances in the lung meridian—the result of "karmic wind," e.g. "lung." Such notions are in line with the *vatas* in Ayurvedic doctrine and the humors in Graeco-Roman medicine.

The experiences arising from habituating with the essential nature of mind, being by definition impervious to change, are of an entirely other order than these blemishes. That said, it is still recognized that the "mind rides the breath," hence the importance of calming mind and breath. As the body-mind complex (the brain being only one component of this rather intricate process) is "realigned" through one's practice (whether meditation, asanas, *pranayama,* Taoist alchemy, or even acts of charity and kindness), these phenomena progress through various stages and upon reaching a balanced biochemistry and physiological matrix subside (e.g. a balancing of the lung).

It is possible that the migrainoid realm encompasses elements that, in other circumstances, are archetypal manifestations and guides into higher realms of consciousness or enlightenment—that the same neural pathways can plummet downward into chaos and psychic disintegration ("unbalanced lung") or radiate upward, through dissolution, into knowledge and revelation. What is a scotoma under one regime is a *tangka* or religious icon and signpost under another (as per the earlier discussion of Hildegard of Bingen). A neural manifestation, put to opposite applications, has not only an entirely different meaning but a different genesis. This suggests the two routes of humankind: evolution and devolution, sometimes mythologized as heaven and hell.

By this iconography, migraine auras can be "suffered" with anxiety, attachment, and denial, or can be embraced with detachment, deep breathing, and simple witnessing and wonderment. Although an aura is not a spiritual signpost as such, it can be enlisted in a meditational practice as if it were and put to developmental use while it is elapsing. The scintillating scotoma, though dominating ordinary activity and making some actions difficult or impossible, becomes a primitive mandala, an opportunity to practice compassion (including self-compassion), dissolution of static in pure mind, and attention to the neural and excitatory basis of all consciousness.

What is of special interest is the linking of the unfolding of these psychospiritual visions with the increased strengthening of the individual's awareness and mental development, and the continual decrease in attachment to all phenomena both external and psychological. The signs of one's progress are not just these visions but also a diminishing of stress and negative emotions such as anger, attachment, and jealousy, together with an increase in detachment, wisdom, and compassion. The ultimate state is said to be one in which the natural awareness remains without distraction in a continuous unbroken stream throughout day and night. During this final stage of internal alchemy, known as "the exhaustion of dharmata," all these visions cease and one simply remains unwavering in a state of pure enlightenment.[40]

Diseases

Let us adopt, for a moment, the premise that chronic diseases are migrainoid, sometimes for purposes of the body-mind reorganization, and sometimes as psychophysical mechanisms (or compensations) beyond our ken. It may be that health is a tiresome balance to maintain and, just as dreams give a daily reprieve from the vigil of consciousness and allow the mind to wander undisturbed in its own elements, diseases actuate highly evolved immune functions from their vestigial components. The organism utilizes the biological equivalent of a "reset" button and, through the process of undoing the aura, renews its holistic balance and capacity for transduction.

Though migraines are disruptions in the equilibrium of the body-mind, unlike pathologies that persist and often worsen or remain static and wear down organs, they run their course quickly, dwindle, and evaporate. They function as diseases, but in benign psychosomatic cycles.

While a true disease may cause actual pathology, it can also inspire a cycle of death and reinvigoration. Like migraines, diseases can be "healthy."

Organisms are well designed by nature; they know what they need and provide it. Countless muddles that challenge them also protect them and keep them functioning day to day. Diseases or neuroses occur when a combination of problems has pushed an organism past the point where it can cope; yet symptomatic compensation is often an initial phase of self-cure. Migraines might then function as substitute pathologies, more ephemeral and less damaging mimeses in place of diseases, filling the systemic requirements for illness while bringing only pseudopathology and, happiest of all, activating a mending process.

If migraines were "real" diseases, they would be lethal ones (strokes or tumors), but they are simulacra and thereby provide a clue to the disease-and-healing mechanism itself: actually most ailments distort and purge along a migrainoid spectrum. There is nothing in the brain-mind-body that is not migrainoid (e.g. imperfectly synergized, neurally fragile/vulnerable, somewhere along a process of working out its structural and energetic harmony, hence potentially discordant); every state is always improving and deteriorating simultaneously, as the organism shifts from moment to moment and state to state, seeking relative equilibrium and maintaining homeostasis.

Self-corrective processes monitor disruptions and find pathways to restore health, to bring the organism *as a whole* back into harmony and function. Day by day, people are assaulted by a virtually ceaseless array of pathological influences, including (minimally) infections, traumas, injuries, depletions of nutrients, allergies, toxins, genetic gaps, and stressors. Homeostatic mechanisms are regularly challenged and downgraded, leading to dysfunction and physical or mental limitations. As internal communication systems among cells, tissues, and regulatory networks begin to break down, the organism is forced to adapt at a less efficient, less maximal level. Pathological conditions cascade in place of corrective integration, and simple maladies start to collaborate on more complex disease patterns, all in the service of finding a new equilibrium.

In order to keep viscera functioning and psychosomatic regulators dispatching and receiving integrative signals, micro-rhythms and minute molecular movements and catalysts throughout the body must constantly establish terrains that allow communication and homeostatic pattern changes. It is not the peculiar symptoms or warps that matter; it is the overall result, which is life and well-being.

The collective pattern allowing and enhancing self-organization operates by deriving a common ground, a base rhythm, an individual holistic strategy. Auras and headaches may well be aspects of such a signaling system, catalysts that upset the degrading elements or ennui of neurovascular, visceral networks, and, while exacting a price in pain, disorientation, and temporary hallucination and blindness, provide the necessary jolt to get a collective rhythm back.

Life is a violent, turbulent process, neither mellow nor antiseptic. Correction is going to hurt, baffle, and dazzle by the sheer lightning-like fire and battle scars of the continuous struggle for existence.

Migraines are thus state changers, disease epitomes, redeploying stray energy without invading organs. Sacks encapsulates this therapeutic cycle: "It may be important ... to consider migraine ... as a complex, dynamical disorder of neural behavior and regulation. The exquisite control (and, normally, latitude) of what we call 'health' may, paradoxically, be based on chaos.... Perhaps this is especially true in patients with migraine, in whom, at certain 'critical' times, the smallest stress will cause a physiological imbalance [in the central nervous system] which, instead of being quietly corrected, leads rapidly to further imbalances, overcompensations, playing on each other, rapidly amplifying, until it reaches that end-point we call 'migraine.'"[41]

In summary, illnesses are maneuvers by the organism to defend itself from damage, restore equilibrium and, ultimately, recuperate vital powers—and some may be more efficient and benign than others. Apparently migraines fall into the salubrious category—self-organizing meta-neural networks using the brain—the "enchanted loom"[42]—as a palette to produce figments for reasons of overall homeostatic organization, and to control gradients of health and illness, sanity and psychosis, waking and dream.

The sense of molestation imbuing a scotoma is also a shamanic emblem for its mode of ritual cleansing and rebirth.

The Evolutionary Basis of Migraine Auras

Mind and body are in constant collaboration creating reality. Although we experience our existence as a smooth wave of consecutive moments and events, it is sustained and regulated by discontinuous neural mechanisms and irregular bursts. Perception is the collective result of synaptic discharges throughout the sensorium, converting molecules, discharging potentials, and assembling a vast bioelectric field in the process.

Reality is not so much an established thing as the surplus or remainder of extravagant aggregates of computations, all involving the binary distinction between zero and one, a cipher that is used latterly by computer chips to turn images and meanings into commodities. Hierarchies of intermittent oscillations have to be synthesized into a single wave in the command structure of the brain. Awareness is, in effect, an organized spasm, a tamed aura. Its pulsation provides the veneer of everyday scenery and cognizance. Tweaks, tremors, and other interferences in it yield dreams, phantoms, and ambiguous phenomena at different levels of autonomy.

Migraine auras encompass a sort of spasmodic hiatus in the feedback loop between mind and matter. The excited neural rudiment takes on a life of its own and gives rise to an intrinsic construct, the scotoma with its artifacts. A break not in the ophthalmic landscape but its substratum of hard wiring and code, it bears startling resemblance to the gibberish that appears when a computer page devolves into the symbols that engender its ordinary viewing option. Most people have experienced an error whereby programming language with its field of ostensibly meaningless symbols replaces a document or image on the screen (or alternately leaves a gap or hole in the middle of a text or image). These collections of signs and cutout blanks replicate scotomata. They speak to a similar mechanism: if underlying code is interrupted or unconventionally translated, the resulting image will be distorted, interrupted, or obliterated. Glitches or gaps on the screen may even evoke an aura because they are so similar to one.

How did the anatomy and structural hierarchies of the nervous systems of ancient land animals and then mammals and primates develop? Were there multiple possible routes to centralized organization of perception and data? Are there different possible "viewing options" for reality? Were there crossroads of arousal and cognition when evolutionary choices were made, perhaps even arbitrarily, in relation to meaning? Do synaptic, binary nervous systems interpreted and ruled by ganglia represent a series of adaptive resolutions concluding in sense organs, neurons, and brains? Are their pathways random or molecularly inevitable? Were there crises along the way, gaps that were mended by patches, chaotic elements that were jury-rigged into workable cellular instruments? Do migraines and their auras speak to these imperfect repairs and conditional modifications? Are they routine pathologies and breakdowns of the sort that must occur in all systems, or do they encompass emergencies and compromises that freed and elevated neural traffic through the ganglia of our predecessors? Are their spasms perhaps even alternate and imperfect "experimental" frequencies of reality?

Though these questions will never be answered, we can at least address them from the premise that migraines once had an adaptive purpose.

If auras and their equivalents have primacy in zoological functions, these far antedate humans and even antedate mammals. Insofar as scotomata are effects of the invertebrate brain—the basal ganglia and brainstem—they are associated with our most primitive chordate and reptilian pathways, including those that are reality-based and distinguish waking and alertness from narcolepsy and trance, especially the sort of trance in which comb jellies and sea squirts spend their entire lives.

The phenomenological worlds of jellyfish, marine and land worms, and mollusks (other than the octopus) are relatively quiescent, preconscious, and passive. These animals sense the environment and respond to it, but they do not "awaken." It took an arousal mechanism cresting in central ganglia, in concordance with other evolving organ systems, to get them darting, pouncing, and snapping with cognitive *oomph*. The catalyst could have been a migrainoid glitch in the brainstem.

Though fanciful, this proposition is not outlandish. Some sort of elemental progenitor of dreams, hallucinations, dreamlike fugues, and other chimeras probably inhabits rudiments of the brainstem— those that are involved in testing of the external world and creature identity. Existential artifacts from disjunctions in these areas would affect the development of arousal and reality, and *vice versa*. Thus, migraines and dreams might have blossomed alongside perception and cognition in their earliest forms—and modern migraines might represent their equally old, vestigial by-products. Their recurrences (or relapses) result in partial sensory distortions (auras), imaginary realities (dreams and trances), and diverse other spasms. Historically, though, before there was a distinction between raw sensation and primitive ideation, when dreams and auras were fused with phenomenological similitude, these artifacts could have played a role in the discriminative emergence of consciousness and its first symboling and abstracting organs—its emerging entelechies. Before auras became perceptual defects, they were proprioceptive utility programs, auxiliary functions of incipient states of conscious awareness.

Imagine some sluggish lizardlike creature. In order to get it active and tactical, the brain has to fire continuous alarms, wake-up calls, baseline alertness. The creature is busy in fits and spurts as it is aroused. Then it lapses back into semi-coma. Millennia later, its primate descendants (like us) are kept awake at the level of cerebral consciousness, by thoughts; we don't need extraneous arousals. But if such an alarm clock were built into the primitive brain, it might well be interpolated through evolutionary phases into far more complicated neural structures, and its old firings might then get integrated into other body-wide homeostases or remain (as well) vestiges of a former preconscious regime.

Migraines might be a lingering window into an archaic phase in which consciousness used positive and negative triggers (patterned gestalts and their negation in meaningless excitation) to discriminate itself from the flood of mere excitation through which it necessarily ascended, jellyfish to worm, salamander to ape. Contemporary scotomata embody to some degree an anomaly or displacement of an original summons—a simple, pedantic, and relatively accessible lesson in the relationship between reality and its neurosomatic artifacts, between what can be organized empirically in a primate and what simply organizes itself randomly and preconsciously in a newt (both of which are essential, in the contrast between the two, for awakening). To a jellyfish in its eternal pulsing, an aura is not a pathology or degradation but, potentially, *a message.*

That is not to say that auras necessarily have an evolutionary function crucial to the survival of our forerunners, only that they are operating at a level of anatomy and consciousness where *other* critical functions arise and they generate activities and actions to be assessed in actual zoological species and events.

Far less devious and challenging than dreams, aura precursors could flag an epochal shift in the areas of the brain associated with waking and alertness, certainly by the stage of marine chordates. Among simpler animals that were their forerunners, archaeo-auras could have overridden former cues and tropisms, meshing sensory input and creating a perceptual field.

Or an aura could be a functionless by-product and figment of such bridges, a consequence of a series of developmental predicaments, anatomical compromises, and their vestigial contrivances to get out of *cul de sacs* in the overall rivalry of environment, anatomy, genetic capacity, and adaptation. There may not have been a perfect solution at a number of points, but emergent consciousness "needed" to move to the next phase or wither. Creatures were not only ready to reality-test, but their revolutionary anatomies made reality-testing critical for survival.

Scotomata and fortifications could be incompletely formed calls to mindedness, early crude harbingers of subject-object discrimination. Adaptive initially as actuators in chordates, fish, amphibians, and reptiles (or as the derivatives and superventions of actuators), they have become stagnant and detrimental in us in whom the arousal/consciousness mechanism has climbed to upper, emerging levels of the brain.

Let us take it from the bottom up: Paramecia and other unicellular zooids are almost solely reactive. Alive but unconscious synapses at a macromolecular level, they subsist in independent pulsations, homologs of cells in more complex mammals. For one-celled entities, a pulsating cell is obviously the whole reality; in multicellular creatures, however, all cellular "realities" are contextual and interdependent as they flow upstream into ganglia. Invertebrates such as clams and worms have been compared by anatomists and embryologists to organs of the mammalian body and lobes of the human brain.

Organismal homeostasis itself is a generalized primitive function that has evolved in stages through the animal kingdom. It is possible that the simpler the animal, the more generalized and migrainoid (or involuntary) its basic movements are. Jellyfish, crickets, ants, bees, termites, etc., have nervous systems that operate in diverse and diffuse waves of unconscious stimulation and activation, many of them collective and transpersonal, as is patent among insects in their hives and swarms.

If subtle triggers akin to those that set ants and bees into collective vegetative activity are dispatched vestigially by the human brain with no utilitarian outlet, they now and again may attain the status of signals and emit sterile beeps rather than acts. If insect behavior is migrainoid in etiology, then a common proto-migrainoid stream of taxes, mimeses, and scotomata might confer fundamental biological meanings as well as a lineage on auras.

Remnants of jellyfish and worms certainly linger in the historical viscera of all creatures that have evolved along their templates. Passive reactions with accompanying secretory and visceral activity recur widely among animals, even ones that maintain in their repertoire very forceful and powerful movements too. Mammals share ancestors with coelenterates, mollusks, and worms. Lions purr as well as stalk and mutilate. Chimpanzees go into trances as well as swing through trees. Humans "freeze" and faint in fear as well fire guns. The cowering of a dog, the arching of a cat, the curling up of a hedgehog, the sham death of an opossum, the changing colors of a chameleon, the rattle of a rattlesnake, even the odiferous squirting of a skunk and the dam-building of a beaver suggest passive, somatically regimented and autonomic aspects of nervous systems.* The light patterns of phosphorescent beetles and fish and the taxes of insects and insect larvae are expressions of a deeply subliminal range of arousal/autonomous trance phenomena. These behaviors are almost like *elaborately externalized migraines*. In fact, the color var-

---

*Such reactions are probably far more diverse and widespread across the natural world than we realize insofar as we have quite limited access to animal psyches.

iegations that creatures display are, at least metaphorically, a somatic counterpart to the kaleidoscopic phenomenology of auras. In that sense auras might be like relics of aboriginal movies inside us of the interior lives of our invertebrate forerunners, as if we were able to see some of the protean processing mechanisms and hierarchical waves underlying the propulsion of an octopus or mental calculations of a starfish. They would represent—in an internal regime—the genetically prescribed behaviors of free-living cells and cell clusters in zooids at large: convulsions, choreas, faints, mimicry, entrancements, noctambulations, photophobias, photophilias, migratory grids, hyper-alertness, low capacity for conflict without resolution, mating dances, web-spinning, hive-making, and so on.

Insofar as the migrainoid world runs from relatively simple spasms and chimeras to dramatic mirages and entire experiential philosophies, an aura is a phase of physiomental integration, not a departure from or rent in it.

Migraine capacity may be a recurrent, vestigial aspect of animal life as a whole, suppressed or subjugated in more conscious creatures. The imaginal qualities of auras demonstrate the uniquely elaborate differentiation and fertile ideation of the human cerebral cortex which makes new use of all sorts of brainstem codes and discharges: it not only receives arousals passively but continues to organize, interpret, and reintegrate them into higher-level concepts, metaphors, fantasies, and phantasmagoria. An aura in a starfish or snake is probably a fleeting buzz or flicker-film, whereas in mammals it becomes embroidered and elaborated by the cortex into pseudogeographies.

A developmental crisis that could be successfully resolved at a migrainoid level in invertebrates because of a *lack* of capacity for further consciousness becomes a hazard again at a different cerebral level when passed on to creatures with immense capacities for totems and meanings. That is, invertebrates and simple vertebrates were not disturbed by auras because their migrainous spasms were so close to their ordinary migrainoid functioning they could use them to mate, swarm, attack, sleep, and awaken.

Having opened the discussion of auras to the history of arousal and neural discharge and the origin of phenomenological reality, I have conjured a possible iconography for experiencing migraines optimistically when they occur. They are not aberrations of healthy mind-body operation; they are the jagged underbelly of vision and thought itself, revealed when the skin is temporarily torn off the landscape and its basis is exposed or—phrased differently—when the normal processes of the nervous system are interrogated at their root.

In that spirit, auras are less unwelcome intrusions than vestigial capacities operating in humans at a localized and superficial level. Their arousal and inhibition waves serve universal biological and psychological codes, but they have been synopsized and condensed over time to minor, contingent disturbances because of our more symbolic and cultural existence. We have no great need for physiological "hallucinations" as arousal or reality devices because we have invented and inhabit a world of intellectual ones, but we do have need for artificial pathologies to heal our burgeoning stress patterns, neuroses, and inner contradictions and introjections. Hence, atavistic motifs have been both marginalized and recovered in us, for they still respond to stimuli in the environment and nervous system, sometimes certainly for reasons of dysfunction, sometimes as somatopsychic compensations and displacements, and sometimes as superfluous but powerful agents seeking new roles and meanings.

In any case, the nervous system cannot drop something so primal and old—and would not drop it if it could, partly because it has already been organized by developmental and phylogenetic precedent and is stuck in our biological mechanism and protocol, and partly because of the instinctual and proto-libidinal priority of such "nostalgic" responses as ingredients—pivots and sutures—in other, higher-level organismic mechanisms. In the context of myriad challenges, creatures must draw on whatever components are accessible and at hand, every day as well as archaeologically, even those that serve no present function and are in fact disabling and maladaptive. Once upon a time they meant something crucial; now they simply *are,* structurally and hierarchically.

At some point biology might find new meanings and functions for them. For instance, they could become the basis for still-developing telepathic or telekinetic capacities. To invoke an infamous neo-Darwinian fable: in a nanotechnological world decades or centuries from now in which ordinary sources of industrial energy have been exhausted, those with a crude but innate ability to act upon molecules directly will have a survival advantage.

What is an afflictive, nonsensical migraine today is once and forever an act of arousal from the lizard/hedgehog sleep of universal unconsciousness. Beyond tomorrow's tomorrows it could generate kineses out of our present waking trance of Stone-Age cybernetic culture and help lead the way into a realm of projective psi, remote viewing, and psychic healing. Earth would have a whole new sensorium, a presently unimaginable internal science, technology, and source of energy; it would be a different planet.

No harm in wishing such! But it probably shouldn't happen too soon or it might yield a world of thaumaturgists and corrupt magicians armed with voodoos and hexes.

The Chaotic and Organizing Structure of the Brain and Nervous System

The new science of chaos, complexity, and nonlinear systems is used to explain self-organizing systems, as simple (relatively speaking) as weather fronts and as complex as cellular integration or cultural activity. Patterned order is somehow implicit in matter. Autonomous semi-symmetrical motifs occur even in inanimate chemical mixtures, giving rise to crude geometrical configurations, one propagating out of another, "circular waves expanding concentrically from a fixed center, spirals that twist outward, clockwise or anticlockwise."[43] Self-organizing whirlpools and rainbows develop harmonic oscillations and proportionate congruities, changing color and self-transforming into more complex systems that dissipate and then reemerge. They evolve and disperse naturally out of one another, as their remote forerunners did in the nebula cloud that gave rise to stars, solar disks, and planets and, at a different scale, oceans in worlds among solar systems and living organisms in at least one of those oceans.

Inherent order occurs everywhere in nature. There is no difference between chemicophysics and psychobiology, between whorling rivulets in a pond and "a wavelike excitation propagating across a sheet of cortical matter."[44] Everything in the universe tends toward implicit self-organization. What the old physicists regarded as linear, static cause and effect—a heat-controlled cybernetic machine—is actually a series of dynamic systems that reinvent themselves out of matter and energy, providing everything in existence, even the arrow of time. The seemingly random cosmos is "an immanent organising intelligence."[45] There is no great device, no automaton, likewise no extrinsic teleology or Maker: "The universe is like a giant brain."[46]

Nonlinear dynamic systems are structured and self-maintained by multiple layers of interconnection and feedback within themselves, for anarchic entropy gives birth to order through—paradoxical as its seems—inherent, unordered multiformity and multiplicity. Every haphazard and partially enclosed system both diverges from and converges into a range of potential states, each of them a summation of its components. These so-called "phase states" are semi-stable distributions of the parameters that they encompass, arrangements of elements that continuously achieve temporary balance through which they express a persistent but fragile capacity to sort, convolute, unravel, then reorganize differently.[47]

Chaotically cohesive systems are maintained by attractors, e.g. anything at all that can hold their semi-stability—their self-generated sequencing or structure—in a nonlinear hierarchical conformation in the absence of any other influence. Gravity and heat are the primal agencies, leading to both structures and boundaries.[48]

Chaos systems wobble and oscillate because they are conserved solely by a dynamic harmonization that could always collapse into disorganization. Not only patterns within natural landscapes and life forms but motifs within cultures are inherently coherent and self-organizing: that is, the mathematics underlying seemingly random animal behavior and demographic and socioeconomic themes, as well as styles of social structure, shelter, art, and dress, when analyzed algebraically, produce unexpectedly orderly graphs that reveal semi-equilibria and patterned shifts of self-organization, roughly congruent from feature to feature. These design elements arise as if from nothing, or from the chance elements of prior systems, and in turn give rise to their successors.[49]

The otherwise mysterious dynamics of somatic, visceral, and psychosomatic phenomena ranging from cardiac rhythms to language are cognates of the partially symmetrical bands across planets like Jupiter and Uranus: vast chaotic meteorologies resolved regionally into regularities, color-banded stripes and oval cyclones within gravitational fields.[50]

Emergent complexity forms the basis of our nervous systems, and it does so while made of mutinous molecules, lieged to entropy and gravity, lassoed into compounds and cells by delicate and volatile biochemical gradients and homeostases, hence under continual threat of disintegration. We are elaborate storms inside semi-permeable membranes. Mind itself is a turbulent active chaos system.

As we discussed in the preceding section, landscapes are fashioned in the brain, not the external world or eye, by dots and pixels that blend like a Monet painting into sheets and scrolls with boundaries in differential relief, recognizable as scenery, landscape, figures, and meanings. Not only are we constructing reality out of serendipitously patterned and ruthlessly geometrized parts, but those elements then maintain their own unruly integrity, as scotomata reveal.

In generating perception and mindedness, chaos/order dances along a cusp, deriving cohesive, sensible patterns out of what *should be* entropy of billions of separate, unconnected synapses. It is listing always toward breakdown into such gibberish. Thus, the entire neural and cerebral enterprise within a creature, like the creature itself, is held in a dynamic semi-equilibrium, organizing cellular potentials, generating patterns out of sensations, landscapes out of nerve firings, philosophies out of electrical and chemical potentials. At any moment, though, all of these might break down into the mud out of which they long ago formed; yet it is that very threat that keeps them healthy, dynamic, and evolving.

Spontaneous self-organization, by its very nature, elicits its opposite: spontaneous self-disorganization. Each continues to disintegrate into and reintegrate from the other out of which it receives constantly shifting energy and structure to renew itself in different forms. The visual components of the nervous system are in states of tenuous equilibrium for the achievement of sight, and their temporary disruption leads to the neural process being perturbed and artifacts (scotomata) being generated; i.e., component pixels rebel and organize new kinds of gestalts and pseudogeographies, restructuring perception and meaning.

An aura is thus a dynamic cycle within the nervous system as a whole, converging upon and diverging away from surrounding dynamic patterns. Like Jupiter's red spot, each scotoma tends toward entropy (inertial feedback and mirage, at least in relation to lucid perception) but is dangled in place by opposing attractors in the cerebral cortex—one pulling vision toward ordinary sight and habitual meaning, another disrupting it into lower-level turbulence. The result is a partial hallucination, an optic artifact.

Using the "kaleidoscopic power in the sensorium to form regular patterns by symmetrical combination of casual elements,"[51] the ocular cortex cannot turn totally anarchic or adventitious—after all, it is a satellite of the pattern-ridden sorting function of the brain; it renews the fragile visual field under preordained attractors.

The scotoma thus forces a coalescence of entropy and geometrized order upon nonparticipating and resistant elements of mind. After it sets them amok around an eccentric attractor, the visual field begins reconstituting itself out of self-organizing mosaics and synapsing hierarchies. The more evolved attractor of the "normal" system pulls itself out of the aura into its established method of synthesizing sensations and presenting consensus reality. Order is temporarily restored; the aura dissipates.

Fractals are geometric epitomes operating within dynamic systems, forms that repeat their own elements at ever smaller scales, engendering complex shapes while compacting their complexities into space. The mathematics of fractals provides modes for analyzing such shapes and their underlying exigencies as means of filling anatomies and landscapes.[52]

Fractalization is a primary physical process in the universe. It is the method by which large, complicated structures made of random elements under gravity fit into the spatial constructs they generate as well as into space itself. Stars, cells, shorelines, anthills, beehives, and nervous systems are all fractal architectures.

The expansion of a phosphene into a full scotoma, the projection of a triangle into a zigzag line and then a series of hexagonal figures with a shining ring inside them, the emergence of a network of sensation "with sudden jerks, 'like frost on a windowpane'"[53] are similarly fractal; they follow the same formal principles as rivers, coastlines, gas giants, the development of intestinal villae from a single villa, or the bifurcation and expansion of a maple tree along a branched pattern from a single sprout. Fractal geometry is a coordinating feature of migraine auras as they arise and propagate, probably responding to the renegade attractor of a neural burst from below the cortex. This attractor fractures polygons into smaller ones, e.g. hexagons nesting tiny hexagons, patterns dispatching self-similar icons, and "radially symmetrical forms like flowers or pinecones, continually unfolding in a constant revelation of themselves . . . before the inward eye, enlarging endlessly in a self-similarity."[54]

Migraines cannot be assigned to a mere mechanical or molecular cause, single relationship, or even a physical failure. They occur for integral dynamic reasons, as static in the nonlinear equilibrium of nervous systems. While it takes an initiating stimulus somewhere along the cerebral hierarchy to trigger an aura, alternate stimuli can converge and agitate the brainstem or other aspects of the neural field enough to incite migrainous (e.g. strident) impulses. This is why, as noted earlier, migraines are both hard to prevent and remediable only at a cost elsewhere.

With the activation of a wave of disorganizing potentials, patterns of excitation and ideational remnants flow through diverse, highly sensitive neural fields, setting off synapses in other waves, which interfere with one another, producing patterns at a minimum of two levels—that of the actual neuron-firing mechanisms in the brainstem into the visual cortex itself and that of the secondary, cognitive organization of those patterned firings into images, ideas, and concepts—the pseudo-landscapes and fractal structures seen by migraine sufferers.

The brain is intricate: "a hundred million cells, twenty cell types, six layers, an infinity of connections both intrinsic and extrinsic [with] action potentials which result from the movement of ions in and out of the cell in a complicated time-dependent manner."[55] You cannot model any particular perception-disequilibrium pattern; you can only hypothesize the generalized potential of many possible nondifferential actions involving neural synapses. "[T]he partial differential equations representing [auras] do not converge to a single solution, but instead diverge and bifurcate into innumerable alternatives."[56]

Reconsidering migraine etiology in the combined context of complexity theory and evolution, we can classify sensory phenomena as gestalts that build upon prior or more primitive matrices of unorganized, lower-level fragments to generate vision, sound, orientation, sensation-continuity, and then reality, language, and philosophy. It is the chaotic, frangible dynamics of synapsing and sorting, embodying an enormous bound charge, that gives neural systems their flexibility and evolutionary potential. They entertain new capacities because they are not rigidly trapped in old patterns or condemned to repeating the same designs and functions. They evolve irrevocably, along with the rest of nature and biology.

Sacks celebrates this neo-Darwinian cortège: "[N]ature 'thinks' in nonintegrable differential equations, 'thinks' in terms of chaos and self-organisation, 'thinks' in terms of nonlinear dynamical equations. . . . Such systems tend to hover far from equilibrium, and it is this far-from-equilibrium position which gives them their sensitivity, their criticality, their capacity to change radically and unpredictably, to generate, to evolve, new structures and forms." They "produce order through fluctuations."[57]

The way mind was put together originally from austere ganglia in marine worms and amphibians (and has evolved over time) recapitulates itself eccentrically and quasi-coherently in auras, trances, hallucinations, and hallucinogenic visions of all sorts. These are generated by the nervous system's refined organized stability and also the various creative instabilities into which it can crumble when disrupted, yet out of which it emerges with new capacities and, over millennial time, new organs, synapses, and methods of classifying information and making consciousness.

Parading through various edge-of-chaos metamorphoses, scotomata are x-ray visions into the once-and-future schema of the brain. By removing key factors from the equation, they reveal how the equation was put together in the first place. By perturbing the image in the mirror, they allow us to see how the mirror reflects distortion and then repairs itself epochally, in twenty minutes. We are looking at the unrefined river of space and time.

Vision and reality cannot be maintained forever. Erosion of the entire system is inevitable—absolute chaos, absolute scintillation, absolute blindness. Every organism, every brain, every reality is on the highway to dissipation and death. A migraine aura is a premonition of this entropic fate but, because it occurs within a vital living system, it is temporarily subdued and its pixels corrected. For a time, order triumphs over higgledy-piggledy. The homeostases of life and integrated vision find a way to restore themselves through molecular micro-movements and cellular regimes. Protoplasmic streaming and hierarchical matrices self-correct and contribute to macro-rhythmic harmony.

Some of the terror elicited by auras may be the premonition that we will dissolve, ego and all, back into the primeval clutter from which we emerged. When balance flirts with disequilibrium and a migraine discharges through the nervous system, we get breathtaking vistas into not only the brain but the electromagnetic field and chemical bath in which we were forged. It is a hint of what it would be like to plummet, like the astronaut in the movie *2001: A Space Odyssey*, down through the cloud layers of Jupiter, into cruel and utter chaos.

The Relation between Physiology and Psychology in the Brain

I have tried to make a story for auras, but it is also worth considering that they have no story, at least no story in words. Dreams have a story—in fact, many stories. Their narratives are spun by the same neural agencies as waking, but without a lodestar of worldly scenery. Commands, trapped within the brain's feedback, draw on bound emotional charge and excitation to weave nonlinear landscapes. Whenever sleep coincides with intrinsic brain activation, external stimulation is barred and internally arising motor impulses are locked in. The reticular system, which regulates the brain's activity by electrochemical showers from deep in its stem, discharges anew onto some hundred billion neurones. As these are strafed with erratic pulses, an increase in acetylcholine and dopamine coincides with a hyperactivation of emotional centers in both the limbic lobes and the zones of the cerebral cortex that integrate emotion with perception.

Conversely, secretion of biogenic amines like norepinephrine and serotonin is inhibited. These aminergic neurotransmitters, originating in the brainstem and terminating in the amygdala, normally modulate forebrain activity: coordination, primary sequencing, and temporal categorizing—that is, by providing a chemical basis for connected memories, logic, critical judgment, relevance, and directed attention, they usher non-synchronous, non-sequential messages into temporal relationships. Without their neuromodulation, simple correlations are not made; normal cognition does not occur.

The consequence of near simultaneous activation and deactivation—acetylcholine enhancement and norepinephrine/serotonin deficiency—is a gated trance state: hallucinations, exotic landscapes, delusions, strong emotions, anxieties, and global amnesias.

Freud assigned dream formation to unconscious wish-fulfillments at tension with modes of concealment or repression from the horror or shame of the wish. Freud's dreams are sublimated networks of instincts streaming through the brain while being translated into imagery: free associations, memories snapped from their temporal context, and "events" hybridized from these streams.

But while forms seek meanings, forms are also expressions of system components and constraints. For post-modern neuroscientists dreams are neither wish-fulfillments nor censored documents but naked improvisations of the brain, its attempts to rationalize from disparate cues, to ease the disorientation and anxiety caused by objectless bombardment.

Migraine auras, originating likewise in the brainstem and involved with similar imbalances of neurotransmitters, may be the *waking* brain's conciliatory response to a chemico-electrical artifact imposed on optical transmission. The exotic shapes of the aura represent an intersection of anatomical and associative options available to the nervous system.

We do not know what auras are because auras are things, not meanings. Clarity of mind and vision flows right up to and around a migrainous wave. Whereas dreams are fusions of meanings and emotive shapes sealed into paradoxical cinemas, auras are sensori-motor phantoms, fugues that are strange, disorienting, and disturbing because they are *not locked in.* They start from a tiny rip—and then cut a slash in fully alert consciousness over which they impose the gauze of their throbbing emblem.[58]

III.
The Treatment
of Migraine Auras

When to Worry and When Not

More Common Migrainelike Diseases

Neurologists and other physicians have discovered no permanent damage or irreversible changes from migraines or their auras. Thus, from the standpoint of allopathic (standard mainstream) medicine, which is generally neither philosophical nor holistic in its orientation, the apparent danger of a migraine is that an overly hasty diagnosis might miss a more serious pathology; i.e., a migraine history should not lead one to minimize *all* discrepancies and variations from normal vision as benign and transient. Since the visual effects of auras represent the passage of abnormal chemistry and electrical distributions through the nervous system and brain, virtually the same artifacts could arise from many causes, some of them quite dangerous.

It is initially important to distinguish migraines from ophthalmic conditions like glaucoma and other deteriorations of sight. Eye diseases that appear to be auras may be evaluated against the following examples:

Corneal edema and acute glaucoma can produce halos or rainbows around lights.

Foreign bodies in the cornea and conjunctivitis-based mucous strands can distort light in a variety of ways.

In the lens of the eye, the development of posterior subcapsular cataracts can generate shining artifacts.

Since scotomata are located in the brain rather than the eye, the likelihood of a neuropathology in the guise of an aura is greater than that of an ophthalmic disease. Just because a person has had migraine auras does not mean he or she could not also suffer from another condition that discharges through similar outlets in the cortex and general nervous system. Migrainelike symptoms mark cerebral diseases like epilepsy, initial signs of Parkinson's, carcinomas, and strokes.

Certain scotomata, visual distortions, disorientations, memory loss, etc., while migrainelike, are not migraines. Some could be symptoms of a brain tumor, angioma, aneurysm (blood-filled dilation of blood vessels), or other malignancy. The following three points of divergence may be signs of serious neuropathology: a unilateral scotoma (that is, a distortion that occurs on only one side of the visual field or in one eye); a static scotoma (that is, a blemish that does not travel across the visual field but remains in one place); a long-lasting scotoma or the persistence of a scotoma in some aspect.

A scotoma should transit across the visual field and be gone in twenty to forty minutes. It might innocently last an hour, but much longer than that, and certainly three or four hours or throughout a day and into the next day, increasingly suggests the possibility of a different condition. (Nonetheless, there *are* occasionally very persistent scotomata.)

Other symptoms that resemble migraine auras but could indicate tumors, blood clots, aneurysms, strokes, or retinal disease include disappearances of objects in the visual field that do not self-change, shift, or get restored; flashing and shimmering lights willy-nilly; glistening bright irregular sparks; distortions, lattices, and blurs that persist and complexify like a distorted trick mirror; or any of these artifacts combined with paralysis, memory loss, fainting, and other stroke symptoms.

In 2005 the American musician Neil Young suffered a persistent migrainelike obstruction in his vision like a broken piece of glass. Under medical examination, this turned out to be an aneurysm.

The flickering of the scotoma closely resembles occipital epileptic discharges. A very brief aura discharge of only a few seconds' duration is emblematic of epileptic attacks. Suspicion of epilepsy or some parallel pathology should lead to testing for correspondence of symptoms with EEG changes characteristic of other seizures.

The aura's cerebral depression wave is close to what might occur from a blood clot.

Visual scotoma-like hallucinations can also be sparked by psychoses, schizophrenia, autism, and bipolar affective disorder.

Drugs like digoxin and clomid can simulate aspects of a migraine aura. Digitalis can induce xanthopsia (yellow vision).[1]

Transient photopsia might indicate a concussion.

Giant cell arteritis can mimic the blindness of the negative scotoma.

The progression of a migrainelike hemianopic scotoma (i.e., a blemish in one half of the visual field of both eyes) may signify a tumor, arteriovenous malformation, and/or focal lesion over the visual cortex or involving its pathways.

On rare occasions headaches with auras mark a subarachnoid hemorrhage. When there is suspicion of this, lumbar punctures are made to obtain laboratory samples.

Floaters

The gelatinous vitreous fluid of the eyes often becomes more liquid and less cohesive with aging, particularly after the age of fifty. One eye at a time—which one yields first depends on a convergence of factors over years—the gel may cave in on itself while peeling away from the posterior retina along a posterior-to-anterior path, yet always remaining affixed to the most peripheral retina. As subsequent rapid eye movements slosh the vitreous fluid inside the eye, it yanks at its remaining attachment to the retina, and the traction can produce brief, benign flashes, especially upon quickly moving the eyes or looking suddenly to one side. If the retina comprised pain-sensitive nerve endings, the effect would be pinprick sensations or acute pangs, but photoreceptor cells indigenous to the retina respond with painless lightning-like flashes, sparks, and/or "scoto-moid" effulgences.

These scintillations sometimes have a compound pattern or "oil-slick" appearance uncannily similar to an abrupt "here and gone" scotoma. Like MAWOHs, they are discharging optically rather than tactilely, hence their aura-like figments. However, a true scotoma not only persists but evolves with dynamic integrity and trails a visual deficit.

A flash that lasts only a split-second in the peripheral visual field is thus likely caused by vitreous traction on the peripheral retina.

Floaters are a more common outcome of posterior vitreous detachment. Their shadows on the retina indicate non-transparent debris in the vitreous gel, the main candidates being red blood cells, white blood cells, pigment, vitreous strands, and retinal tissue. Hard floaters are not luminous or dynamic; they do not change shape or oscillate. Their motion clearly differs from that of scotomata: drawing momentum from their position in the undulating gel, they continue to be propelled even after eye movement has ceased, shooting pendulously beyond the eye's tracking. Scotomata, by contrast, scrupulously escort eye movements.

When the liquefying vitreous separates from the optic nerve, it remains attached by a complex translucent disk of coalesced collagen fibers and fibrous astrocytes. This artifact, known as a Weiss ring or Weiss' ring, is usually visible as a large, multiplex floater. It may occasionally be mistaken for a migraine aura or, more likely, create motifs in the visual field that make the person more susceptible to auras.

Floaters and Weiss rings are neither dangerous nor treatable, since surgery would put the retina and optic nerve at risk.

Other kinds of scotoma-like flashes can be caused by retinitis, retinal microemboli (small occlusions) or, more seriously, retinal tears, which also may suddenly release a large number of floaters from intravitreal hemorrhaging.* Note: if an eyeball is gently displaced by a finger, a retinal feature will move with the displacement whereas a cortical one like a scotoma will remain in place.[2]

Very Rare Migrainelike Diseases

Other diverse, uncommon conditions are sometimes conflated with auras or scotoma-like motifs. This is usually because their neural elements discharge into the same pathways and mechanisms. Throughout this book I talk about visual distortions, paresthesia, cognitive deficits, etc., in the context of migraines, but these are not themselves the core migraine, merely its expression by symptoms. Those somatic trajectories are available to wide-ranging conditions that are not migraines.

Amaurosis fugax (transient monocular blindness), ocular hypoperfusion from atherosclerotic constriction of nutrient arteries, cerebral venous thrombosis (blood clot within a blood vessel) with cerebral infarction,† vasculitis, Ménière's disease (inner-ear vertigo and ringing), saturnine encephalopathy (alteration of brain structure from lead absorption), mononucleosis, Epstein-Barr syndrome (a herpes virus that can cause mononucleosis and some carcino-

---

*This is the signal instance in which floaters are not trivial but a by-product of a more serious eye trauma. Accompanying a host of new floaters, pigment or blood in the vitreous is a sign of an actual retinal tear in about seventy percent of patients with posterior vitreous detachments.

†Infarcts are zones of cells (necrotic tissue) perishing from deficiency of local blood supply.

mas), porphyria (genetic deficiency of the enzyme for making heme, a component of hemoglobin, leading to sensitivity to light and hallucinations), multiple sclerosis, spinal tuberculosis, neurosyphilitis (syphilis of the central nervous system), and lupus anticoagulant all can generate migrainelike effects at times, but usually these "auras" accompany other telltale symptoms.[3]

The German poet Heinrich Heine (1797–1856) suffered from migraines in his twenties: objects vacillating in his vision and taking on a grayish, silvery coloring, also transient palsy of two fingers in his left hand, muscular weakness, right-sided paralysis, and episodic blindness and double vision. This almost certainly indicated a serious pathology: chronic neuropathy (degeneration of the nervous system) or a form of syphilis.[4]

As a rule of thumb, the closer an event is to the artifacts and timing of migraine auras as described in this book, the more likely it is to be an aura. However, some physicians differ substantially from this viewpoint. Donald M. Pedersen, writing in the *Journal of Family Practice,* adopts a conservative position—that if there is *any* doubt about a migraine aura, a full medical exam should be undertaken. He gives a range of options and diagnostic techniques for tracking down nonmigrainous and pseudomigrainous visual distortions: "Underlying organic disease must always be considered . . . if the history does not fit or if the neurologic examination is abnormal. A completed tomography (CT) scan and magnetic resonance imaging (MRI) are necessary to exclude a mass or lesion, and MRI should be performed if a venous thrombosis is suspected (e.g. in a postpartum woman with new-onset migraine equivalents). A hematologic evaluation might include a complete blood and differential count and partial thromboplastin time. A vasculitis panel would include erythrocyte sedimentation rate, rheumatoid factor, antinuclear antibody titer, and serum protein electrophoresis. The cardiovascular evaluation includes electrocardiography, echocardiography, and possibly cardiac angiography. If extracranial carotid narrowing is suspected, noninvasive ultrasound Doppler can be utilized; however, complete carotid evaluation requires cerebral angiography. An electroencephalogram is needed if a seizure is suspected."[5] Though all of these would seem to apply to a small percentage of cases, some doctors automatically check patients with migraine auras for other causes.

"MR angiography can be used to diagnose vascular malformations," writes Timothy C. Hain, a Chicago-based physician specializing in dizziness; "MR venography can be used for sagittal sinus thrombosis. MR also may detect low-pressure type headaches, tumors, as well as [postpartum] *Chiari malformation*. Fortunately all of these are [also] rare."[6]

He adds that a prolonged aura (greater than sixty minutes), especially in the context of white-matter cerebral lesions, could be indicative of mitochondrial myopathy, antiphospholipid antibodies, systemic lupus erythematosus (SLE), multiple sclerosis (MS), and cerebral autosomal dominant anteriopathy with subcortical infarcts and leukoencephalopathy (CADASIL).[7]

Mitochondrial myopathy is the name for a class of genetic defects in the protein-producing mitochondria that process food into energy. Among its symptoms are epilepsy, poor balance, fatigue, and migraine-like headaches and seizures with visual impairment.

SLE is a serious autoimmune disease occurring primarily among women and at three to four times greater frequencies among African Americans and African Caribbeans. It attacks multiple organs with widespread vascular lesions from the failure of normal antibody responses.

CADASIL is a hereditary condition affecting the muscle walls in small blood arteries, causing brain infarcts, strokes, and dementia, and is almost always fatal ten to twenty years after its effects appear.

Among its diagnostic symptoms are classical and common migraines with severe depression.

In unusual cases implying any of these (for genetic or other reasons), "persons with prolonged auras should get coagulopathy testing—to look for lupus antibody, anticardiolipin antibody, proteins C and S, and factor V Leiden."[8] Skin biopsies to test vascular smooth-muscle cells may be necessary in cases of suspicion of CADASIL.

White-matter lesions in MRIs and/or in subjects with prolonged auras or severe headaches, even in the absence of other pathologies, usually lead to physician recommendations of prophylactic measures.[9]

Mainstream Remedies and Therapies*

The Best Remedy Is No Remedy

People are deluded by a technologically experimental and invasive corporate medical system for which the guiding priority is to discover biophysical loci and develop products for them, not to cure actual diseases in sick people. It is an institutional bureaucracy first, a clinic or hospital second. Modern medicine is dominated by an unacknowledged commodification of not only pharmaceuticals and

---

*I have written extensively on health, disease, and medicinal systems elsewhere and, since it is impractical to graft much of that material here, in notes through the remainder of this book I will cite other volumes of mine that deal in much greater detail with theories of cure and treatment options. These works, regardless of their original publishers and titles, have been reissued by North Atlantic Books in revised and updated editions as *Homeopathy: The Great Riddle* (1980, 1993, 1998); *Planet Medicine: Origins* (1980, 1995, 2000, 2005); *Planet Medicine: Modalities* (1980, 1995, 2003); and *Embryogenesis: Species, Gender, and Identity* (1986, 2000). *Embryos, Galaxies, and Sentient Beings: How the Universe Makes Life* (2004) was not previously published or revised.

"medical time" (physician and hospital resources, etc.), but pathologies and cures as well such that, though few participants realize it and most would be appalled to step outside the system and observe what has happened, the goal of professional healing is more commercial than therapeutic.* Under this regime Sacks accuses the "migraine ... establishment of 'medical overkill' and patient exploitation."[10] Some doctors have even carried out surgeries in hopes of ending migraine attacks, though fortunately not (to our knowledge) cranial or cerebral ones. Gallbladders, teeth, tonsils, uteruses, and ovaries have all been eviscerated as possible migraine instigators, especially when there is a second excuse to remove them.

Sacks is convincing in his plea that surgery of any sort "has no place in the treatment of migraine,"[11] adding that there is often temporary, rebound relief from surgery itself, no matter what is removed. Since we are dealing with multi-level, nonlinear networks, the shock of incision and organ extraction is bound to have an activating effect on sensitized mechanisms, and that may be an explanation for alleviation. Migraines are changeling conditions in dialogue with anatomy and psyche, so they tend to retreat in the spirit of displacement or conversion without fundamentally vanishing. They turn into unconscious or differently pathologized forms of the same thing. Symptomatic relief from surgery is usually either transitory or deals some other unpleasant equivalency for the migraine.

[Although general surgery is not advisable, an exception may be insertion of cardiac devices or catheters to close the patent foramen ovale or PFO, a practice that has been adopted in the early 2000s to treat some migraines in the United States and Europe with promising results. This would only be viable in instances where PFO closure coincides with chronic migraines, a correlation in an estimated

---

*See *Planet Medicine: Origins,* pp. oovii–36, and *Planet Medicine: Modalities,* pp. 519–537 and 551–578.

3 million of the approximately 28 million American migraine sufferers. This obscure agency, unrecognized through decades of medical research, came to light because of strokes from blood clots that passed through the open shunts of patients who happened to have migraines too. Closure of this valve in many stroke victims eliminated their migraines too—as approximately half of those with abnormal PFO openings suffered migraines as well. Now PFO valve diagnosis (and closure, if indicated) is available as a migraine treatment option.[12]]

It should be noted that none of the many holistic and complementary options is reliable or universal in its application to migraine auras either. This is particularly true when alternative medicines are just ecologically "correct" forms of allopathy, using herbs, manipulations, or needles in place of drugs and surgery, but still targeting and attempting to reverse a particular locus of cause and effect.

Since migraines almost always resolve themselves promptly and have a compensatory and purgative role in the homeostasis of body-mind, they probably cannot and should not be squelched routinely. If there is marginal justification for remediating something, treating it runs a greater risk of doing harm rather than good. Any aggressive therapy is likely to have more deleterious side-effects than "smart bomb" impacts on the symptoms. Those side-effects may actually curtail or delay self-healing, regardless of any symptomatic benefits such as muting of headaches. Since migraines do not wreak enough damage to require intervention, iatrogenic (physician-caused) pathology from an attempted remedy may be far worse than the disease, as will be clear from the complications of many of the most popular migraine drugs listed below.

When alternative treatments are most holistic and least aura-specific, they are most beneficial, if not curative, because migraines are systemic in nature, have emotional and psychosomatic components, and cross many organ boundaries. Getting healthier and stronger in general usually means fewer headaches, fewer auras, unless the migraines are necessary to discharge some trenchant toxicity or malaise. Removing migraine symptoms, conversely, can introduce complications and pathology.

Remember, one aspect of the potential curative power of migraines themselves is their tendency to form representation and replacement cycles with peptic ulcers, hay fever, psoriasis, motion sickness, Crohn's disease, panic attacks, menstrual syndromes, neurotic guilt cycles, and various other migrainoid-pattern pathologies. Whenever the migraines occur, the other condition or conditions are lessened or disappear altogether. When the migraines retire, the other conditions return (see p. 80). This would suggest that the body-mind experiences a *fundamental equivalence* between migraines and other maladies that is not evident objectively, as the organism makes a biopsychological choice of how to express and heal disease processes more fundamental than any of their symptoms.

To one degree or another, the option of treating or not presents itself to every migraine-aura sufferer. If an aura has a function in the overall regulation of the organism, then that function should not be needlessly interrupted or interfered with. In fact, an old axiom of medicine recommends not removing any obstacle until it is clear at least what the "obstacle" is protecting.

Sacks mentions a patient who experienced periodic Sunday-afternoon migraines until he prescribed an ergot drug for him. The migraines and premonitory auras ceased but were replaced, at least in terms of Sunday scheduling, by fresh attacks of a sort of asthma that had ceased entirely years earlier to the patient's relief.[13]

In support of letting migraines elapse naturally and not enlisting drugs to abort them, Sacks offers this additional narrative:

"A middle-aged professor, of fiery temperament . . . tends to get classical migraines on Friday afternoons, following his inspired and stormy teaching sessions. He has scarcely time to rush home from these before scotomata and other symptoms make their appearance, followed within minutes by violent hemicrania [one-sided head pain], nausea, and vomiting. If these symptoms are *endured,* they run their course and resolve in three hours, leaving a wonderful sense of refreshment, and almost of rebirth. If, on the other hand, they are *aborted* (as they may be by ergotamine, exercise, or sleep), there is a persistent malaise throughout the entire weekend. Thus this patient is presented with a *choice:* to be violently ill for three hours, and then perfectly well; or to be vaguely ill and wretched for two or three *days.* Since realizing his situation, he has given up the use of all abortive measures, finding a severe but brief migraine altogether preferable to a mild but greatly extended one."[14]

The possibility that migraines and their auras are fundamental, necessary utilities of the nervous system and/or latent solutions to bioemotional crises raises the consideration of whether they are not *always* best left to run their brief course and dissipate on their own. Scotomata may be debilitating and uncomfortable—for instance, when a migraineur is lecturing to an audience and a person in the group turns into a Picasso clown, or when she is driving and another car's glaring back window puts a blind spot on the highway—but they are still self-resolving, whereas their so-called "cure" may lead to other, less benign problems.

Hindu post-structuralist blogger Madhuleema Chaliha lauds the alchemical power of a sacred disease: "The bad part of a migraine is, without a doubt, the migraine itself. The good, and the most beautiful, part of it, however, is what happens after it has passed away. Unlike a medicine that leaves a bad taste in the mouth, a migraine almost always goes away leaving a strange feeling of wholeness inside my mind. It is the most destructive poison that I know of that contains with itself the seeds of regeneration."[15]

As an ancient and uncivilized part of our metabolism, migraines may in fact be more medicines than diseases. Unlike contemporary miracle drugs or novel "painless" technologies, migraine "healings" psychosomatically foreshadow the Pomo bear shaman who roams the woods with a goal to wound as well as heal (in fact, each is working at a level that does not make a distinction between the two).*

In nature the most primitive episodes are often the most profound and powerful ones, eliciting forces to which we have no access otherwise. We might not willingly enter their domains—but nature doesn't give us that choice. It reaches into its repertoire, which goes back to simple oscillating cells and spasming jellyfish, and calls upon their diffuse vibrations. Cures of arousal and dissipation lurk in that abyss and transmit its primacy and alchemy.

Prevention

One of the most effective alleviations of migraine auras is simple prevention of circumstantial scotomata before they occur. A person might begin by learning how to direct his/her attention away from fixation points or triggers. Biofeedback, breathing, and visualization exercises all offer possible retraining methods. Sunglasses might help in a few instances, although they are not a panacea and have secondary effects on the eyes (for instance, curtailing exposure to the nutritive aspects of sunlight).

Biofeedback is a laboratory modality developed in the 1960s to teach subjects to alter normally involuntary bodily functions such as blood pressure, heart rate, and brain activity. Reduction of migraine symptoms was one of its initial objectives. A biofeedback machine picks up electrical signals from the body (for instance, tightening of a muscle) and displays them in the form of a flashing light or beeper. This signal serves as both information and "reward" to a

---

*See *Planet Medicine: Origins,* pp. 86–87.

subject who then tries to breathe, relax his or her muscles, and change habitual responses to tension in a way that can be tracked and displayed by the machine. The wiring collects biofeedback from the body and makes it intelligible so that automatic behavior can be addressed with awareness. The goal is to improve mind-body function, and this is accomplished by changing the machine's readings, not by controlling sensation in a conventional manner. For whatever reason, people can respond more effectively to an extrinsic light or sound than to their own remote, undefined feelings. In a sense, biofeedback proposes to achieve the same results indirectly and clinically that yoga and meditation accomplish experientially. Hustvedt describes a relatively successful encounter with such an appliance:

"No relief came until my neurologist had exhausted all his cures and I was handed over to a psychologist who taught Biofeedback. I then trained with a strict behaviorist,* a man who belittled Freud (to my chagrin) but who nevertheless had a cheery disposition. For nearly six months, I was connected to a machine every week that measured my ability to relax. For a person who began this medical adventure in a state of near panic, I eventually became an expert at it and no longer need the apparatus. This technique does not prevent either aura or headache. It helps to tame the symptoms after the fact, and I can almost always lessen my pain now through deep relaxation."[16]

Many other alleviations are matters of common sense. Not eating during an attack is an obvious precaution, even if one is already at a meal. If an aura is incited by candlelight in a fancy café and one proceeds to try to consume the food they have ordered, despite a lack of appetite, this can make the nausea worse.

---

*Yes, in a gentle way biofeedback is behaviorist.

Ice-packs on the forehead are successful with some people's symptoms. Hot showers, which alleviate other forms of headaches, tend to make migraine ones worse, but not in everyone, and they have been known to soften visual auras slightly. Almost any form of massage—Swedish, craniosacral, acupressure, Rolfing—is helpful.

Famously migraine sufferers retreat into dark, quiet places and seek sanctuary from any exacerbating noise or brightness, including normal levels of conversation and indoor lighting. Migraines should in fact be an opportunity for withdrawal and hibernation, until the scotoma and/or headache have passed. Sacks describes his favorite migraine clinic: the only medicines are aspirin and a pot of tea, and the patients are directed, with a few quiet words, to darkened cubicles with beds.[17]

Improving lifestyle will reduce incidence and/or severity of migraines in some people. Dietary precautions include avoidance of highly processed, fatty, spicy, overly salted, and sweetened foods, and any foods in binge or semi-binge fashion. Balancing diet with one's metabolic type is another option.

If a particular substance seems to incite or aggravate auras, one might consider eliminating it from her diet or medicine chest. Dairy products, alcohol, and fermented foods are all migraine suspects. Cheeses, coffee because of its caffeine, chocolate (which also contains caffeine), and carob are generally contraindicated. Corn, nuts, avocadoes, yeast, citrus fruits, and many spices can be selective migraine triggers.[18]

Though caffeine can paradoxically help prevent migraines, overuse leads to rebound headaches. As far as cheeses go, the more ripened or aged, the more risky—cottage and American cheese are *not* known to trigger migraines, while cheddar, mozzarella, parmesan, romano, bleu cheese, brie, etc., have been identified as occasional culprits. Wine contains not only alcohol but nitrates, and these have multiple negative health effects including migraine sensitivity. Red wine is considered to incur the highest risk. Nitrates are commonly used in preparing foods such as bacon, sausages, hot dogs, and packaged lunchmeats, and these should be regarded as potential hazards.[19]

MSG (monosodium glutamate) is a famously identified migraine co-factor, and it should be avoided in all its guises: autolyzed yeast extract, hydrolyzed vegetable protein, or even the deceptive "natural flavoring(s)." Cheap Chinese restaurants and fast-food franchises routinely use MSG, but even glitzier establishments have been known to elect it as a simple, feel-good flavoring. MSG hides out in soy sauce, yeast, yeast extract, meat tenderizers like Accent, salad dressings, hot sauces, and seasoned salts.

A number of medications can cause migraines, even some drugs that relieve headaches in other instances. Medicinal triggers include the afore-mentioned nitrates (in such forms as Nitroglycerin and Isordil); Zantac (an antacid); hormones such as birth-control pills and estrogen-replacement therapies (see below); Lupron; Provera; cold capsules and decongestants; and foods and medications with caffeine in them (as noted). Scintillating scotomata have been triggered, either directly or indirectly, by the use of oral contraceptives, confirmed by aura cessation at their discontinuation.[20]

A startlingly high percentage of female migraine-aura sufferers never saw a scotoma before they began taking hormones at menopause. There are many reasons why a woman might terminate hormone replacement therapy, and migraines are probably not the major one; nonetheless, some migraines begin with the ingestion of hormones and cease when they are stopped.[21]

Beneficial activities range from hiking, running, biking, and sports to martial arts, do-in, and yoga, and encompass consciously deeper breathing and exercise on a regular basis, consistent sleep patterns with sufficient sleep, and avoiding overwork.

It is not so much a matter of eliminating migraines directly through a particular dietary component or mode of behavior as introducing elements into the field of body-mind in which migraines breed from interactions of multiple factors. If single elements are changed or synergized in different ways, the complex grid in which headaches and auras spawn might be repatterned such that symptoms become less frequent because they do not have sufficient tension or co-factors to generate themselves.[22]

Other, non-dietary trigger factors for migraines (and auras) that could be experimentally avoided are air travel, becoming overheated, strong smells (especially perfumes), unusually distinctive tastes, and (as noted often) bright lights and noisy venues.[23]

Emotional health is obviously important too. Whatever migraine auras are or are not, they are usually indicators of stress and conflict. Dealing with deep-seated life problems and trying to reduce aggravation in common-sense ways might also eliminate migraines. Since auras play an emotional and symbolic role in the psyche, the deeper one goes into their own "issues" and life, the more likely one is to influence the level from which artifacts are generated.

Placebo Effect

The body-mind is a complicated, cohesive colloid that is electrically unified and subject to multiple gradients of induction and control. Many conditions can be altered at points that are far removed from the targeted symptom. Even popularly prescribed pharmaceuticals are consistently successful in treating pathologies in situations for which there is no chemicophysical rationale. The organism has countless enzymatic, hormonal, psychosomatic, and other triggers, any of which could have a cascading effect reaching virtually any organ or process in a person. Elimination or addition of a food or drug from one's repertoire might lead to a cessation of migraines for arcane reasons. A particular pharmaceutical, though not intended for treatment of migraines, could have a therapeutic result because of its impact on other systems and their secondary or tertiary hormonal effects.

Because migraines are erratic and might lessen or stop altogether for a variety of obscure reasons, their decrease or cessation may not be confidently attributable to any one practice, treatment, or drug. It is virtually impossible to tie a particular medical action to a change in migraine symptoms, so one must proceed on a premise of enhancing overall well-being and capturing the aura in the widest net. In contrast to allopathy, one doesn't have to know why a "holistic" modality works, as long as it does. Even placebos are powerful drugs; i.e., the suggestibility of the mind with its capacity to affect biochemical and metabolic systems is oft-times sufficient. Since migraine auras are psychosomatic phenomena, placebos have a real possibility of cure—and without the long-term toxic side-effects of "real" drugs!

Psychosomatic participation in a substance that one believes may aid in a condition, quite apart from any biochemical impact of the substance, can itself spark a therapeutic response. The formula works because of a positive biofeedback loop created in the organism by a combination of the medicine itself, visualizations and feelings related to it, events triggered by interaction between the two, and feedback among these and differential levels of the system.*

Placebo effect is not quackery. It can in fact be the most powerful cure of all—thought and belief are magical, instantaneous forces. They function negatively as voodoo curses in witchcraft; for instance, in tribal societies where the pointing of a bone or maleficent spell may cause someone inexplicably to die. It is no wonder then that a beneficent projection may result in a mysterious cure. In fact, physicians regularly participate in "placebo" projections, both curative and pathological, unintentionally and unconsciously all the time.

---

*See *Planet Medicine: Origins,* pp. 211–224, 379–465, 497–508, 520–526, and *Planet Medicine: Modalities,* pp. 579–604.

Without intending it, they "successfully" wish health or project hexes on their patients, and the consistent ability to facilitate beneficial transference may distinguish a good doctor.*

Drugs and General Allopathic Approaches [24]

There are *no* standard drugs targeted for the aura components of migraines and few even semi-reliable ones for headaches or the greater migraine complex. With its willy-nilly expressions, migraine is a moving target with multi-tiered effects that are almost impossible to specify. While some drugs appear to be migraine-effective, these also raise suspicions of placebo effect or transient symptomatic improvement.

In general, Americans consume pharmaceuticals indiscriminately in search for "miracle" cures, treating their body as if it were a machine or chem-lab experiment. They pay little attention to the actual effects of drugs, which target a specific organic reaction by either inhibiting or catalyzing it, nor to other effects of this reaction on processes in the body that are assimilating new molecules and enzymes. They also give little thought to the consequences, either short- or long-term, of the biochemical interactions of so many pharmaceuticals and their by-products. People are fundamentally transmogrifying who and what they are, often without significantly improving their health.

A surprisingly diverse range of allopathic pharmaceuticals has been tried on migraines in a scattershot approach over the years, and new drugs continue to be developed and tested. There are problems with all of these:

• No "successful" migraine medication works consistently or with all patients. Migraines have quite different causes person by person,

---

*See *Planet Medicine: Origins,* pp. 167–185, and *Planet Medicine: Modalities,* pp. 122–131.

and it is futile to treat a differential complex as if it were a unitary event.

• Drugs are evaluated solely by their capacity for alleviation of a particular symptom—and discarded from pharmacopoeias if not routinely successful in that circumscribed task across diverse populations. Large pharmaceutical companies have little interest in formulas for individualized and idiosyncratic kinds of conditions because they cannot generate nearly the same levels of profits from them as by mass-producing drugs for universal use.

• Drugs may have quite different effects depending on the route of administration—by pills, liquids, aerosols, suppositories, capsules, or injections. Some migraine medications gained their reputation in emergency rooms where intravenous (IV) delivery is common, but they are ineffective when administered orally.

• Almost all—in fact probably all—migraine medicines have more serious side-effects than the symptoms they are treating. Headache sufferers might protest this characterization on the basis of the severity of their pain but, however baneful, migraines are still not pathological, whereas migraine-attacking drugs well may be. In essence, in medicating migraines, physicians and patients are choosing to treat a brief functional or clinical disturbance rather than an actual disease, and probably on a symptomatic basis. Yes, some allopathic medications curtail auras and/or headaches, even for good in some patients, but those cures are subject to the qualifications mentioned elsewhere in this book.

• Because of the chronic nature of debilitating migraines, there is a danger of drug dependence and addiction from repeated reuse, meaning increased tolerance to pharmaceutical effects, withdrawal symptoms, consumption for longer or more often than recommended, alteration of lifestyle to accommodate drug activity, and secondary inability to manage without the drug (even apart from dependence on it for migraine alleviation).[25]

• There is poor biochemical explanation for the action of any drug on either headaches or auras. Explanations for migraine drugs are conjectural at best. In many cases doctors and pharmacists have no idea how or why a particular molecule "works." Drugs are prescribed with opposite intent, for instance both to raise and lower serotonin levels. Neural stimulants (like amphetamines) and sedatives (like Valium) address seemingly quite opposite migraine elements.

• The brain is far too complicated to treat along unilinear (or even multilinear) pathways. Researchers have learned more about cerebral function in the last ten years than they did in all previous centuries, as they have gone from mechanical to electrical to neuro-transmittal to complexity models; yet they still only speculate about how the brain operates. Plus, medicating the brain can result in unplanned neuropsychological complications.

• Paradigms change with scientific and intellectual fashion, whereas mechanisms in nature remain the same. The switch from psychosomatic to biochemical explanations for a range of psychological and borderline psychophysical conditions during the 1960s represented a revolution in both psychiatry and internal medicine. Whether for good or ill is a matter of opinion and will probably remain so for years to come. Not only was Tourette's syndrome transformed almost overnight from a psychological disease with an emotional etiology to a neural disorder that is chemical in cause and treatable solely by drugs, but innumerable neuroses, psychoses (including schizophrenias), phobias, states of depression, and anxiety disorders were increasingly addressed pharmaceutically instead of psychotherapeutically. It should be no surprise that migraines were included in the switch from a psychosymbolic approach to a technological biogenetic one.

• Pharmaceutical companies do not develop migraine cures; they develop medicines for a variety of other uses, and then a few of these are discovered subsequently to have effects on migraines, usually because a person taking a drug for another purpose reports that, whatever the intended effect of the formula, it helped their headaches. When many people make such a claim, word gets around and doctors begin prescribing the drug "off-label" for migraines. Sometimes an explanation will be confabulated; sometimes the establishment accepts "mechanism unknown."

Classes of drugs that were originally designed for the treatment of epilepsy, high blood pressure, hypertension, anxiety, or some other pathology have limited success with migrainous symptoms and are now considered migraine medicines even though the basis of the effectiveness is a matter of speculation. A migraine drug *per se* is almost an oxymoron.

Additionally, drugs for a range of psychological and physical conditions—including poor digestion, constipation, insomnia, asthma, mood disorders, etc.—in individual cases dampen migraine susceptibility. Most psychotropics and mood drugs have been reevaluated at one time or another for migraine use. It is uncertain whether any of these has done more than temporarily suppress one or another trigger and thus somewhat disable the migraine mechanism.

Migraine pharmacy has enlisted adrenaline, nicotinic acid, antihistamines, diuretics, analgesics, amphetamines,* and sedatives

---

*Amphetamines probably have a worse reputation than they merit, at least by comparison to dirtier drugs with more serious side-effects. Originally synthesized in 1887 in Germany as a treatment for narcolepsy, amphetamine works in a manner similar to other migraine nostrums, acting on serotonin receptors while indirectly stimulating release of dopamine and norepinephrine from nerve terminals through a reuptake channel. Speed and crank may create social problems, most of them albeit secondary to the drugs themselves, having mainly to do with economic and political overreactions to them. Their medicinal effects can usually be dozed off with a night or two of good sleep, a reprieve few of the other, more unforgiving migraine (and recreational) drugs offer.

(Librium, Valium, etc.). The major groups of medicines like ergots, triptans, NSAIDs, etc., have all crossed over from other application to migraine status. Gabapentin is presently a popular off-label migraine prescription.

• Since it is the headaches that are almost always targeted (nausea secondarily), my discussion of pharmaceuticals will address the migraine complex in general and specify the rare instances when a drug has reported success with visual auras.

The first class of drugs to be applied extensively to migraines—now pretty much obsolete—was ergots. Too toxic for ordinary therapeutic use until it was isolated in ergotamine in 1918, ergot is a fungus that infests grains. In different recipes it was used historically to hasten labor as well as to treat headaches and Parkinson's disease. Ergot has hallucinogenic properties, represented (perhaps unintentionally) by rainbow-like pills. For patients with adverse reactions to ergot, belladonna (deadly nightshade), an atropine and an antispasmodic and anesthetic, was a substitute (occasionally in combination with ergot and/or phenobarbitol), though by a different biochemical logic.

Ergotamine tartrate (marketed as Wigraine) had the most pre-1960 success for severe migraines. The *ex post facto* supposition was that it adjusted serotonin levels in the blood and dilated restricted blood vessels. Ergotamine can be introduced orally, by injection, as an aerosol, or in a suppository—the oral form being the slowest (several hours) to take effect, thus not very useful for migraines in progress. If ineffective, it can be repeated in a half hour, but then three days must pass before it can be taken again. Isometheptane (Midrin) is a less commonly prescribed ergot drug with almost identical application. Catergot (a mixture of caffeine and ergot) and DHE (dihydroergotamine) are older drugs, though the latter has been made reavailable in a nasal spray (Migranal).

Serotonin (5-hydroxytryptamine or 5-HT) is a neurotransmitter synthesized in the central nervous system and gastrointestinal tract. Plentiful in the bloodstream, it is forged from the amino-acid tryptophan by a variety of enzymes. Its activity in the body is even more complex and nonlinear than most substances, but it is assumed to play a key role in mood fluctuations (including bipolar disorder), anxiety, appetite, and sexuality (by tactile sensitivity and emotional empathy). Recreational drugs such as MDMA (Ecstasy) and cocaine, and many antidepressants inhibit 5-HT reuptake in presynaptic neurons, recycling or metabolizing it and thereby altering transmission over synaptic gaps.

There is no agreement as to the precise role of serotonins in migraines, as the clinical effects of drugs directed at them do not actually correlate with the theories behind them. For instance, if the premise is that there is too little serotonin in the body, then taking a tricyclic should have an effect in hours, but it usually requires at least three weeks. The upshot is that, as noted, some drugs for migraine relief lower serotonin levels, while others raise it. Any migraine relationship is probably not a matter of linear quantity but a differential aspect of serotonin deployment and timing taking place somewhere in the central nervous system well removed from initial serotonin engagement.

Ergot derivatives are quite broad in their agencies, thus have more significant side-effects than triptans (see below). They should not be prescribed in instances of circulatory and coronary disease or for pregnant women, and in about ten percent of cases they cause nausea, vomiting, drowsiness, and faintness. The list of recommended abstainers includes those with liver, heart, or kidney problems, hypertension, cerebral or peripheral vascular disease; women pregnant or lactating; and those using vasoconstrictors, 5-HT1 agonists, the beta-blocker propranolol, nicotine, and macrolide antibiotics (produced by actinomycetes).[26]

Methysergide (Sansert) was introduced early in the 1960s and initially seemed to have success in the treatment of migraine, but Sacks implicates it as a dirty drug with dangerous side-effects, [27] and it is currently banned in the United States. It must be stopped for one month every six months when used, and its impact on the kidneys is such that regular CT scans of the renal organs are recommended after the first year. It has also been implicated in reduced circulation. Joan Didion writes: "[O]ne migraine drug, methysergide, or Sansert, seems to have some effect on serotonin. Methysergide is a derivative of lysergic acid (in fact Sandoz Pharmaceuticals first synthesized LSD-25 while looking for a migraine cure), and its use is hemmed about with so many contraindications and side-effects that most doctors prescribe it only in the most incapacitating cases.... When it is prescribed, [it] is taken daily as a preventive...."[28]

Caffeine was an early popular migraine medication, as it stops spasms in the blood vessels—it also stimulates urine flow. Caffeine is still worth trying as a damper, though (as discussed above) it can cause headaches similar to those that it treats.

Aspirin* can alleviate the force of a headache without unwanted side-effects (except for occasional upset stomachs). Discovered in 1829 with the isolation of salicylic acid from willow bark (which was employed widely in a medicinal context long before its action was understood), aspirin combines analgesic, anti-pyretic, and anti-inflammatory properties and works partly by inhibiting cyclo-oxygenase, a critical enzyme in prostaglandin synthesis. Though it exists only for microseconds, prostaglandin, a hormonelike fatty acid, generates enzymes involved in the production of messenger molecules that operate during inflammation. Among other attrib-

---

*Aspirin contains caffeine and is a NSAID (see pp. 181–182).

utes, aspirin also reduces platelet aggregation that may play some role in the vascular strength of a headache.

With breakthrough discoveries about neurotransmitters in the 1950s, researchers arrived anew at the viewpoint that an anti-serotonin drug might be successful in treating migraines insofar as the condition was coincident with abnormal serotonin levels. Even assuming a serotonin factor in migraines, there are now more than forty identified neurotransmitters, and serotonin receptors fall into three distinct families; thus medicating requires a more discrete and nuanced approach. Nonetheless a whole SSRI (selective serotonin reuptake inhibitors) armamentarium of drugs has been put forth for migraine prevention, with emphasis on headaches: fluoxetine (Prozac), Paxil, Zoloft, Celexa, Lexapro, and Luvox.

A more pure serotonin antagonist and vasoconstrictor, sumatriptan, was introduced in the late 1980s, with some reported success, probably in constricting the microcirculation and inhibiting the firing of the raphé nuclei and trigeminal pathways via 5-HT1B and D receptors in cranial blood vessels, effecting their constriction while inhibiting inflammatory neuropeptide release. Now there is a host of triptans available, all of them fairly expensive but spottily reliable for not only the headache and nausea aspects of migraines but other forms of tension headache. Initially administered subcutaneously during an attack, triptans became available in pill form, nasal sprays, and sublingual preparations, the spray often working the fastest, though it leaves a bitter after-taste.[29]

A new triptan drug, rizatriptan (Maxalt), is generally prescribed in a dose of 10 mg. sublingually and is also considered faster-acting. Almotriptan (Axert) is a marginally less expensive version of the same substance (doses of 12.5 mg.). An even more recent formula, frovatriptan (Frova), approved for use in migraines *with* as well as without auras by the American FDA in November 2001, is regarded favorably because of a long (26-hour) half-life; its recommended dose is 2.5 mg. Sumatriptan (Imitrex), originally given by skin injection, can now be introduced twice a day in pill form (50–100 mg.) but is not considered effective in children. Eletriptan (Relpax) also has quick action when taken orally (40 mg.) but is robust enough to have its use restricted by physicians. Other triptans include zolmitriptan (Zomig) and the slower-acting but longer-lasting naratriptan (Amerge), assimilated in doses of 2.5 mg., respectively. Amerge is used preventively as well as abortively for migraines, especially menstrual ones.[30]

Myocardial infarctions are rare triptan side-effects, esophagal spasms and chest pains more frequent (five percent of patients). Overuse of triptans can lead to rebound headaches. Triptans are off limits for those with heart trouble or blocked arteries, with small infarcts showing on MRIs, with white-matter cerebral lesions, and for those who have taken an ergot medicine, Sansert, or MAO inhibitors (monoamine oxidase-inhibiting antidepressants like Marplan, Nardil, and Parnate) within at least twenty-four hours. When strokelike symptoms are present or during cluster migraines (which coincide with higher risk of heart attack), triptans are also not advised.[31]

Amitriptyline (Elavil), an inexpensive tricyclic antidepressant, has a decent track record for migraine prevention, probably via serotonin channels. Its initial dose is 10 mg. at night, and this is enough for some people; the more common effective dose, though, is 50 mg. It takes two to six weeks to have an impact. Its side-effects are dry mouth, sleepiness, and weight gain, and it has more serious consequences in some people with heart-block or urination problems, pregnant women, and those over the age of sixty. Related drugs include nortriptyline, doxepin, and protriptyline.

Periactin (Cyproheptadine) is a preventive serotonin-related migraine medicine in children, with the side-effect of weight gain.

It is a cholinergic antagonist, i.e., countering sympathetic bodily functions that cause dry mouth, a racing heart, constipation, and general heat.[32]

The levels of another neurotransmitter, dopamine, may also be manipulated for migraine relief. Naturally produced in the hypo-thalamus, dopamine is a neurotransmitter and hormone that acts on the sympathetic nervous system, increasing heart rate and blood pressure. It monitors the flow of information from the frontal lobes to other parts of the brain (its mesocortal pathway), influencing memory, attention span, and problem solving. As part of the basal-ganglia motor loop (its nigrostriatal pathway), dopamine helps the brain regulate smooth, controlled movements. Decrease in amount can lead to Parkinson's symptoms. Dopamine is also considered the "reward chemical" of the brain and its release plays a role in pleas-ure from sex, food, and certain recreational drugs.

Dopamine blockers include Haloperidol (Haldol), Flunarizine (also a calcium-channel blocker), Domperiodone, and Metoclo-pramide. They all have unwelcome side-effects. Droperidol is used occasionally as a dopamine blocker for migraine nausea, but it can have life-threatening cardiac aftermaths.

Bromocriptine, a dopamine agonist used sometimes to treat Parkinson's disease, has been reported in treatment of menstrual migraines.

Migraine nausea has also been treated with dopamine-related phenothiazines like Prochloropromazine (Compazine), Thorazine, and Stellazine, as well as Phenergan, Reglan, and Tigan, but all of these have unwelcome consequences too.[33]

Originally insecticides, the phenothiazines were used to tran-quilize patients diagnosed with schizophrenia and other psychoses, and their neurological and emotional damage validates their her-itage. In recounting the drugs that were prescribed for her migraines during a year following her attack in Paris, Hustvedt dryly remarks: "I saw several neurologists and took a number of medicines, including Inderal, Elavil, Mellaril, and Cafergot, none of which helped me. I was also hospitalized for a week and given Thorazine, a drug that made me feel like a turtle—a soft body encased in a brittle shell. . . ."[34]

Calcium-channel blockers reduce the force of contraction of the myocardium of the heart (their negative inotropic effect); many of them retard electrical conduction, lowering the heart rate by blocking the voltage-sensitive calcium channel during the plateau phase of cardiac action potential (their negative chronotropic effect). This means that cells contract (with less calcium), blood vessels are dilated, and their peripheral resistance is decreased.

Verapamil (Calan), an L-channel calcium blocker, is used for migraine prevention and has been shown to be somewhat effective in one-sided migraines. It is given in 124 to 240 mg. (roughly the patient's weight) per day (standard release). Once the regime is begun, the drug's influence takes about two weeks to kick in.

Diltiazem is another calcium-channel blocker with less of a track record.

Calcium-channel blockers can cause constipation, lowered blood pressure and, in a small number of users, heart palpitations, all indications to stop using them. They should not be used in concert with beta-blockers or in pregnancy but are safe for patients with high blood pressure or asthma.

Other calcium-channel blockers such as nicardipine and sublingual nifedipine are apparently of little utility with migraines, though some authors recommend the latter as a good migraine-abortive drug.

Flunarizine, available in Europe and not the United States, combines calcium-channel with dopamine blocking in one pill and thus has a broad advertised range.[35]

Beta-blockers such as inderal, propranolol (also used for high blood pressure), timonol, atenolol, metaprolol, and nadolol (Corguard) are prescribed for migraine prevention in doses of roughly 60 mg. in the morning or twice a day. Beta-blockers thwart the action of epinephrine and norepinephrine on beta adrenaline-activated receptors throughout the body (heart, bronchi, pancreas, liver, muscles, peripheral blood vessels), thus dampen the sympathetic nervous system and lower heart rate and blood pressure.

These drugs are generally calming but risk side-effects such as hair loss, and they shouldn't be used in patients with asthma, depression, heart failure, diabetes, or while taking verapamil or undergoing allergy shots. Some beta-blockers—Lopressor, Toprol, and atenolol (Tenorman)—are selective, affecting the receptors only in certain organs, while others such as inderal and nadolol are nonselective. Atenolol should not be used during pregnancy.[36]

Not surprisingly, anticonvulsants have been prescribed for migraines. Oxcarbazepine has had occasional usefulness in trenchant cycles but is not FDA-approved for this application. A related drug, carbamazepine (Tegretol), has had little or no utility.[37]

Gabapentin (Neurontin), originally certified as an epilepsy drug, is an anticonvulsant the use of which has been expanded off-label to a variety of ailments as diverse as fibromyalgia and panic attacks. According to Hain, this medicine "does not affect Gaba-b receptors or other commonly studied receptors. It may nevertheless increase glutamate-dependent Gaba synthesis and it also binds to the calcium channel." Neurontin makes people sleepy and occasionally dizzy. It has been associated with weight gain.[38]

Sodium valproate or valproic acid (Depakote), prescribed for general migraine prevention in a dose of 250 mg. three times a day, is also recommended for auras. It is possibly a Gaba-enhancer, though it is not at all clear how it works. It should not be taken during pregnancy or by women of child-bearing age unless they are also on birth control.[39]

Divalproex sodium is another antiepileptic drug adapted for migraine but has side-effects of weight gain and hair loss.

The anticonvulsant Topiramate (Topamax), administered in doses of 25 to 200 mg. a day, enhances Gaba, while inhibiting glutamate receptors and sodium and calcium channels and, to a lesser degree, carbonic anhydrase. Getting higher marks than most migraine drugs, it is reported to reduce headache frequency by 40 percent. Not only does it not contribute to weight gain but it can aid weight loss. It may induce unpleasant skin sensations with no apparent cause, nausea, forgetfulness, and it leads some people to have trouble locating words in their mind and in a few instances has been implicated in severe depression.[40]

A newer drug, Zonegran, has many of the same characteristics as Topiramate (inhibiting carbonic anhydrase while contributing to weight loss) but is migraine-untested.

Buproprion (Wellbutrin), another newer drug (but of unknown mechanism), has been tried with modest results for cluster or chronic headaches and associated symptoms.

Lamotrigine (Lamictal), a formula also with an unknown mechanism (possibly anti-seizure), has been used off-label as a preventive for headaches and vertigo and has been mentioned passingly in relation to auras.[41]

In the latter part of the twentieth century, a group of non-steroidal anti-inflammatory drugs (NSAIDs) was introduced for the symptomatic treatment of migraine.[42] Based on their forerunner aspirin, they include naproxen, tolfenamic acid, mefenamic acid, acetaminophen, ibuprofen, flurbiprofen, ketoprofen, mefanamic acid, Alleve (a naproxen brand), and Tylenol (an acetaminophen brand). These alleviate pain and fever in low doses, and inflammation in higher doses.[43] Depending on which enzymes they hinder, they have mixed results and varied ranges of side-effects, usually at least stomach upset. Tylenol with or without codeine is reported to be somewhat less effective than aspirin and may be addictive. Ultram is sometimes effective. Fiorinal (with aspirin) and Fioricent (with Tylenol) add butabarbital to the mix and may be addictive. They can also cause rebound headaches.[44]

Naproxen is considered relatively safe for pregnancy. Cox-2 inhibitors (including Celebrex) reduce risk of stomach upset but increase that of heart disease.

A red-letter warning: NSAIDs taken in too large amounts can cause kidney and liver damage.[45] A study conducted over six years at twenty-two settings revealed that 42 percent of 662 liver-failure patients tested positive for acetaminophen poisoning, a much higher percentage than for any other factor. Twenty-nine percent (275) of those died, many from suicide after the toxic effects set in. Acetaminophen, a billion-dollar industry from Tylenol sales alone, is now interpolated so widely, both generically and in combination with other drugs, that people accumulate it in their systems without even being aware that they are ingesting it. In fact, of those with liver damage, 48 percent had taken acetaminophen unintentionally.[46] This is a textbook example of a cure that can be worse than its disease: try to improve your mood and get rid of headaches and joint pain, and end up contaminating your liver with toxins and needing a transplant.

Steroids (steroidal anti-inflammatory drugs) were originally developed for the treatment of arthritis and rheumatoid arthritis and then were found to help asthma in the same patients. By the same line of reasoning, they have been used for relief in cases of acute migraine but have limited effectiveness for any other migraine application. They also have unhappy side-effects, well-documented in the sports pages.

Expensive angiotensin-II receptor blockers are used for hypertension and lowering blood pressure and have been tried in migraine when all else has failed or with patients who have toxic reactions to other medications. Angiotensin-II is a peptide maintaining blood volume and pressure. As a vasoconstrictor, it increases blood pressure by compacting arteries and veins, including those in the head. It also works on receptors in the brain to stimulate thirst and desire for salt and releases a hormone that causes the kidneys to retain sodium and release potassium.[47]

Among the newest migraine drugs, ACE (angiotensin-converting-enzyme) inhibitors like candesartin and lisinopril hinder the creation of angiotensin-II from angiotensin-I, thus reduce vasoconstriction and lower blood pressure. Mainly used for hypertension, they apparently play a role in headache prevention.[48]

Botulinum-toxin injection (Botox) is used to paralyze temple, forehead, and neck muscles in order to remove wrinkles, but it has reportedly lessened migraines among those treated (e.g. less frequent headaches and reduced vomiting). There is no explanation, and placebo effect is possible. Some people desperate for migraine relief have tried this method.[49]

Drug treatment is usually a matter of how comfortable a patient or doctor is with simply allowing migraines to continue. According to Hain, "For those who have had more than two severe headaches/month and in patients with complicated migraine (migraine with stroke-like symptoms), a daily medication may be worthwhile. These are generally highly effective (about 75% effective), but do require daily regular use. Examples are amitriptyline (Elavil), Corguard, Depakote, Inderal, Klonapin, Nardil, Sansert, verapamil (Calan, Isoptin). These drugs seem to work via several pathways: some are beta-blockers (e.g. Inderal, Corguard), some are calcium-channel blockers (e.g. verapamil), some work via mysterious routes (Depakote,

Nardil, amitriptyline, Klonapin), and some work through serotonin pathways (e.g. Sansert)." He "usually starts patients with verapamil, and proceeds on to try propanolol and then amitriptyline should verapamil be ineffective. Topamax is also a good alternative."[50]

Among drugs used for related ailments but apparently ineffective or contraindicated for migraines are acebutolol, clomipramine, clonazepam, clonidine, indomethacin, nicardipine, nifedipine, and pindolol.[51]

In conclusion, standard physicians rarely treat, let alone help, any but the most serious migraines, and few doctors welcome return visits from patients after giving a migraine diagnosis. It is no surprise then that alternative practitioners, who counterpoise treatments *with* the energy of diseases, are petitioned for relief. Most alternative medicines are holistic; that is, there is not a specific remedy or technique to match a complaint. Instead, the patient is treated for his or her overall symptom complex, metabolic and psychosomatic state, and emotional and physical vitality.

Alternative Medicine and Migraine Auras

Herbs and Natural Medicine

The herbal treatment of migraines and auras differs from their pharmaceutical treatment more in philosophy than biochemistry. After all, most commercial drugs are based, to one degree or another, on indigenous remedies from throughout the world; thus, in many instances a pharmaceutical substance is, at root, a traditional medicine. Conversely, some herbs are quite potent and have toxic, even lethal, side-effects rivaling the strongest chemical drugs. Differences between herbal and pharmaceutical remedies run along the following lines:

Herbs are most often (but not always) prescribed on a holistic basis to improve overall health, and they influence an underlying predisposition in its expression across many organ systems; whereas drugs are prescribed on the basis of a particular symptom complex and address the complex's effects explicitly while (often) conferring other syndromes. When herbs are employed with the intent of symptom alleviation, it is only in the context of *overall* improved health, and target organs are rarely treated at sacrifice of pathology to non-symptomatic tissues. By contrast, drugs are utilized with the single goal of eradicating a targeted symptom, almost regardless of the cost to other tissues or effect on overall health. Yet molecules are promiscuous and do not obey any prescription for their activity, traveling everywhere in the organism and making whatever bonds nature requires.

If pharmaceuticals have unfortunate side-effects, the only publicly recognized issue regarding these is whether they are dangerous enough to cause the drugs to be banned from the market, i.e., whether they will kill enough people or make enough people sick to create liability for their parent company. Drugs are thus manufactured primarily to make money for corporate shareholders; their therapeutic benefits serve their financial goal, which is what inspires people to invent and synthesize them—not every experimental scientist and doctor in every instance but as an institutional framework for their overall development and manufacture.

Herbal remedies, on the other hand, comprise generations, often millennia, of empirical—not laboratory—evaluation, mostly among tribal peoples. Having no purpose other than the treatment of sickness and realization of health and well-being, these remedies emerged from symbolic landscapes in traditional societies which sought harmony with the universe—with nature, gods, and ancestors. Medicine men and women would not trade relief in one organ for damage to others, as they were striving for holism as a societal and ritual commitment.

Herbs are prepared to treat a person in the cosmos, thus are magical in design. They are especially promising for migraine-aura treatment by comparison with pharmaceuticals because both the disease and the "drug" are operating on a holistic basis. When viewed retroactively in a microscope or spectroscope, that holism may turn out to have been accurate biochemistry (many pharmaceuticals, as noted, originated from research into the virtues of traditional remedies).

Additionally, herbs are mostly decanted from vital botanical or zoological substances (and occasionally unprocessed minerals) and drawn in a raw, infused, or tinctured form that maintains or even enhances their innate properties; whereas drugs are synthesized from dead, artificial chemicals and combined in complex, nonbiological formulas. Allied with foods and nectars, herbs often have a secondary nutritive and energizing effect by contrast to drugs, which are unassimilable foreign elements in the body—deputized intruders, immunity dampeners.

Another key factor is that herbs are selected by homeopathic as well as allopathic principles. This means that they often initially intensify symptoms, as they are meant to elicit—not suppress—an inherent immune response. They are directed at a core disease through its constitutional and characterological dispositions. By contrast, pharmaceuticals are almost always delegated allopathically, with the goal of inhibiting or killing off recognized symptomatic vectors. Of course, herbs can be symptom-suppressing, and pharmaceuticals can occasionally be isopathic (as in the case of vaccinations or injections used in the treatment of allergies), but they are almost never homeopathic.*

I will discuss the homeopathic treatment of migraine auras in

---

*The difference is that isopathy treats a pathogen with a form of *itself* whereas homeopathy treats a pathogen with a *different* substance that incurs similar symptomology.

the next section; for now it is worth noting that most substances developed herbally can also be diluted and then potentized for homeopathic use. The homeopathic potency may have effects akin to its herbal infusion, varying only in subtle ways, but it also may have radically different effects on the organism and disease, bearing little resemblance to its material tincture.

From a biochemical standpoint, homeopathic medicines are for all intents and purposes nonmolecular (as we shall see), whereas herbs are preparations of common molecules. The homeopathic metamorphosis of a substance, if successful in affecting the organism in ways concordant with its herbal cousin, is often metabolically slower, deeper acting, altering more organs long-term, and also less toxic with fewer side-effects—but this is not always true, and the opposite can also obtain. Since a homeopathic preparation is a different chemicophysical entity from an herbal one of the same substance, for it to have roughly the same effects would mean that those effects somehow persist across a fundamental boundary in nature and a change in vibration.

While discussing herbs below, I will emphasize substances that are most often administered herbally, i.e., by herbalists who are not usually homeopaths. For my homeopathic compendium that follows, I will select substances most often prescribed in nonmolecular micro-doses by homeopaths with no herbal training. As it turns out, all the herbs for migraine have equivalent properties in homeopathic form—none of them require qualitatively different herbal and homeopathic applications.*

As individualized rather than common symptom complexes, migraines and auras are diagnosed and treated nonlinearly in each

---

*By contrast, the nonherbal supplements and minerals listed below are probably not translatable into homeopathic equivalents.

person. Because of this and the sometimes antithetical allo-pathic/homeopathic properties of substances in herbal preparation, the range of herbs that *could* be used to treat auras is encyclopedic, probably exceeding 90 percent of all natural substances. In these circumstances I will pick a few plants and minerals that particularly address migraine symptoms, though many others (beyond easy con-jecture) may be effective for atypical sufferers.

To know that an herb has been successful in treatment of migraine auras, there are two benchmarks: are the auras reduced or eliminated and, more important, is the person's overall well-being enhanced? The latter is what makes herbal remedies beneficial when they succeed: pharmaceuticals mostly ignore the second.

As is the case with synthesized commercial drugs, most herbs used for migraines are directed at the headache component. The one exception is chelidonium (*Chelidonium majus,* or celandine), a bright yellow poppy with deeply divided leaves, yellow-orange juice and, like opium, a medicine partly because it is a nerve potion and psyche-delic. Though a headache remedy, chelidonium is prescribed for classical migraines and MAWOH. It is additionally proferred for nonvisual auras and migrainous pains in general—neuralgias, aches, facial tingling, etc.—plus a spectrum of nonmigraine ophthalmic problems. Interestingly, the word "chelidonium" comes from the Greek name for "swallow" (rendered in English as "of the swallows") because, in ancient times, these birds were observed rubbing the plant on the eyes of their chicks, ostensibly to make them able to see better. This provides the plant's other names: swallowwort and kenning wort (seeing plant).

In traditional Chinese medicine, migraine is called "gallbladder headache" because it is associated with gallbladder stagnation, gallstones, and intermittent pains along the gallbladder meridian. According to Taoist principles, meridians are embryogenic channels associated with a key organ on their course (by which they are identified). By "embryogenic" I mean that they encompass basic trajectories and potentials of ontogenetic cellular activity, tissue differentiation, and boundary formation during fetal development. The meridians retain some of this vitality as well as an original capacity to distribute both illness (caused by stagnation or overstimulation) and medicine (in the form of revitalization or sedation by herbs, needles, and less common methods such as cupping or moxibustion*). Both diseases and their cures follow their channels.

The gallbladder meridian travels from the gallbladder (which stores bile from the liver) up the spine, about an inch to either side of it, along the neck, over the occiput, down both sides of the head and temples to the cheekbones and into the eyes. According to this etiology (which is reminiscent of the Greek humoral interpretation of auras), migraines are caused by sluggish, hence thickened, bile backed up from the liver into the gallbladder and gallbladder-liver ducts and from there into the bloodstream, causing an inflammation that emits a damp rising heat from the swollen liver and gallbladder into the scapula region and head.[†] To mediaeval herbalists, who went by the doctrine of signatures, chelidonium's yellow-orange color represented jaundice from liver disease. This does not necessarily make migraine a hepatic rather than cerebral ailment but instead suggests that dynamic relationships among tissues achieve energetic expressions that transcend our names for organs. In any case, by this theory migraine is a circulatory ailment affecting the gallbladder meridian holistically and energetically, all the way from the gallbladder to the brain and eyes.

Chelidonium's reputation at large is cleansing and decongestive, particularly in regards to the liver. The seventeenth-century herbal-

---

*Cones of burning herbs (see *Planet Medicine: Origins*, p. 356)

[†]For a rebuttal of this argument, see the acupuncture section, pp. 207–208.

ist Nicolas Culpepper boiled chelidonium root with a few anise seeds in white wine to break up liver and gallbladder obstructions, alleviate jaundice and itching, and heal lingering sores. This potion was also dripped into eyes to cleanse them from "films and cloudiness that darken the sight."[52] By melting bile obstructions and drawing mucus from the bloodstream, liver, and lungs, medicines distilled from chelidonium dissolve paroxysms that would rise into the head.

The plant's virtues are best transmitted by a tincture made from the flower within minutes of being picked, a general prerequisite of herbal medicines, which depend on the living qualities of their substances. Chelidonium is toxic in large material doses, so is often diluted or prepared homeopathically (see below). Sanguinaria (bloodroot), an equivalent herb, is tinctured almost solely in homeopathic form.[53]

Feverfew (both *Tacacetum parthenium* and *Chrysanthemum parthenium*), a plant containing a chemical called parthenolide that is grandfathered into the U.S. regulatory system as a dietary supplement, has the best long-term reputation among herbalists for treatment of migraine. The guess is that, by stimulating the circulatory system in general, improving bloodflow, and prolonging bleeding time, it dampens one of the co-factors in auras. Feverfew is a component of almost all commercial herbal migraine remedies.

Concentrations of parthenolide in capsules are more effective than ground flowers or teas, the latter because of their molecular loss from dilution and vaporization. Dried leaves require at least 125 mg. to be minimally effective, and contact dermatitis at this level elicits mouth ulcerations in 10 percent of users. Although most doctors consider feverfew a placebo at best, it contains a potent chemical and should neither be mixed with NSAIDs, steroids, or anticoagulants nor given to pregnant or breast-feeding women.[54]

The herbal forerunner to aspirin, white willow bark *(Salix alba)* is still used for the treatment of headaches. Because 1–5 liters of tea must be consumed for allopathic effect, it is of questionable utility, especially since, in that quantity, it contaminates the liver. Homeopathic benefit from low dosages may help some people.[55]

St. John's wort *(Hypericum perforatum)*, more commonly employed as an antidepressant, has been introduced into some herbal headache formulas. As with many other migraine remedies, its role interacting with various other ingredients and enzymes is unknown, but it apparently has success in a small percentage of migraine cases. It should not be taken in combination with an SSRI, as these will interact to elevate serotonin levels dangerously. *Hypericum* can also cause hypertension and photodermatitis.[56]

Garlic cloves—whether consumed whole, in concentrated pills, or crushed and sniffed—have long been a candidate for improving migraines, though in truth there are few ailments for which garlic is not recommended. The adenosine component of garlic slows platelet clumping in blood, so garlic is a circulatory purgative and anti-clotter, as well as an antiseptic and general cleanser of the respiratory system.[57]

Butterbur *(Petasites hybridus)* is a newly popularized migraine herb. A root and/or leaf extract of this plant is recommended for the headache matrix but with an apparent reduction in auras too. Butterbur contains the molecules petasin and isopetasin, zooactive plant lactones with widespread biosynthetic routes and cascading enzymatic effects including inhibition of some metabolic reactions. Its active molecules tend to decrease hypertension and depress both cardiac contraction and intracellular calcium (Ca_2). Like chelidonium, butterbur is utilized for decongesting the gallbladder meridian.[58]

Wood betony improves digestion, nerve signaling, the vertigo of motion sickness, and overall neural and cerebral functioning, having both a relaxing and strengthening (tonic) effect. Used to treat strokes in ancient times, it was administered immediately afterward to limit brain damage. It is also favored for eye spasms and bodily paralysis. Considered to have a grounding influence, wood betony was the herb of choice in mediaeval times for demonic possession and visions and has been rediscovered in a modern context for inconsolable paranoia following UFO abductions.

A mint with a vanilla flavor, best picked before flowering, betony is prepared as a boiling-water infusion of dried leaves or as a tincture of chopped herb macerated in brandy.[59]

The dried root of black cohosh *(Cimicifuga racemosa)* in tea or capsule form is not a red-letter migraine alleviator, though it is widely used among American Indians for many female conditions and has been dispensed successfully for menstrual migraines. A relative of buttercup, cohosh unbinds fluids and muscles, improves blood circulation, and alleviates headaches associated with cerebrospinal congestion or meningeal swelling. Also called black snake root or rattle root (because its seeds make a sound like a rattlesnake), cohosh gets its English name from an Algonquian word relating to pregnancy, as it was used to hasten childbirth.[60]

Although more migrainoid than migrainous in its applications, a blend of black cohosh (3 parts) and wood betony (7 parts) with black hawthorne (5 parts) and pedicularis (15 parts) has been effective (at 10–15 drops daily) in treating nausea, nausea-related headaches, and general faintness associated with auras and aura after-effects.[61]

Agrimony, a small woodland herb that grows in different varieties with similar medicinal properties throughout Eurasia and North

America, has been more popular among native Indian shamans than Western herbalists. A member of the rose family, agrimony is prepared as macerated leaflets in brandy or an infusion that has a raspberry-like taste simultaneously sweet and sour. Like chelidonium it is a gallbladder-meridian medicine, relaxing arterial flow into and out of the liver while balancing arterial and venous channels. When ascending forces along the gallbladder meridian are a migraine co-factor, agrimony is one remedy of choice, though usually second to chelidonium. Agrimony affects many other organs as well: intestines, particularly when there is bleeding in them; kidneys when circulation is constricted; lungs in cases of bronchitis and asthma; female reproductive organs when ovulation is erratic or impeded; and the circulatory system when it is contaminated with toxins. By extension, agrimony is used for speeding the healing of welts, wounds, and burns; balancing intermittent fevers and chills; and dissolving anger.[62]

American blue vervain, a favorite medicine of Eastern Woodlands Indians, is considered more potent than European varieties. All parts of the plant—flowers, seeds, leaves, and roots—are used to make mauve-colored tinctures or bitter teas. An antispasmodic, vervain is a red-letter remedy for epilepsy; it is also useful in reduction of fevers and alleviation of symptoms of menopause. Vervain and willow have been brewed together with surprising success when all else has failed in treating prolonged migraines.[63]

The bog-growing root of blue flag *(Iris versicolor)* is a blood cleanser and hypoglycemia remedy that flushes sugars from the liver. It is prescribed for faintness, nausea, and headaches and also used as a laxative. The homeopathic version is favored.[64]

Coenzyme-Q (or ubiquinone, one of the quinone molecules found extensively in plants) is a vitamin-like substance that has been somewhat effective in reducing nausea and migraine frequency. In fact, the therapeutic effects of ubiquinone are both extensive and mysterious and could certainly extend to migraine auras, as quinones are one of the sources of energy production in all cells of the body.

Discovered and isolated in 1957 and enlisted for a variety of medical uses since the 1970s, coenzyme-Q is a powerful antioxidant that neutralizes harmful free radicals; it has been used for cardiovascular ailments since the recognition that many of those with congestive heart failure have a deficiency of this coenzyme in their cells.

A white powder available in caps, capsules, wafers, and tablets, ubiquinone is recommended in amounts from 50 to 200 mg., with 100 mg. three times daily being a popular dosage, but it becomes effective in some people (for instance, those with Parkinson's) only in ranges around 1200 mg. per day. There are occasional side-effects of heartburn, nausea, dizziness, and non-migraine headache, and it is not recommended for those taking anti-clotting or diabetes drugs.[65]

Riboflavin (vitamin B2) in a dose of 400 mg. a day selectively reduces migraine frequency, but only in common migraines, those without auras.[66]

Petadolex, a formula of 50 mg. of the herb butterbur and 2 mg. of riboflavin, is recommended for both migraines and hay fever. It is unusual for a medicine to be effective in two different conditions, but it is also possible that the twinned ingredients strike at the core of a deeper migrainoid complex. Taken three times daily, Petadolex has shown migraine improvement of at least 50 percent in 71 percent of responders [as per *Neurology 2002*; 58 (Suppl. 3): A 472].[67]

Magnesium as a dietary supplement, usually in combination with calcium (or intravenously injected), has prevented migraines in some sufferers, probably because of the complicated role played by magnesium in brain chemistry, but there is no direct explanation or track record of consistent success. One M.D., Alexander Mauskop, claims a startling reduction in migraine symptoms from a recipe combining feverfew with doses of riboflavin and magnesium for a "triple therapy" preventive approach. The trademarked supplement Migra-Lieve contains these ingredients in percentages recommended by Dr. Mauskop.[68]

In aromatherapy, plant essences are imbibed mainly as scents, the presumption being that odors from concentrations of pure substances catalyze enzymatic activity via olfactory lobes of the brain,* as both migraines and aromas ravel in the cerebral hierarchy. Some essential oils for treatment of migraines—with their scents and generalized applications—are rosemary (rich sweet evergreen aroma, used for cramps, as a heart tonic, and internally to cleanse blood), peppermint (cool menthol aroma, used for fevers, congested sinuses, agitated thoughts, and internally for nausea and vomiting), anise seed (licorice aroma, used for heart palpations, erratic breathing, vomiting, nausea), coriander (sweet, woody aroma, used externally in rubs for arthritis and rheumatism and kneaded on the temples for migraine), ginger (sharp, pungent aroma, used for memory and general headaches), marjoram (sharp, sweet, dry aroma, an antispasmodic used for increasing circulation by dilating arteries, and for digestive spasms, flatulence, anxiety, insomnia, and overactive sex drive), and lavender (sweet, purifying aroma, an antispasmodic, decongestant, antidepressive, and antiseptic).[69]

An "outsider" migraine treatment is the eradication of *Helicobacter pylori* bacteria in the stomach and digestive tract. A study (see

---

*See *Planet Medicine: Modalities*, pp. 447–451.

p. 109) indicates significant improvement in twenty percent of sufferers who had their "bad" bacteria eradicated.[70]

If one did not want to hazard the side-effects of strong antibacterial drugs (among them, wiping out "good" bacteria as well), two or three daily doses of probiotic capsules containing healthy bacteria might increase their populations at the expense of *Helicobacter*. Anecdotal evidence suggests lessening migraine-aura frequency from probiotic use.

One other, quasi-naturopathic technique worth mentioning: From mediaeval times until relatively late in the development of modern medicine in Europe, blood-letting was commonly prescribed for migraine. It was a popular treatment for many ailments, and migraine in particular seemed to represent an excess or superfluity of blood and vapors and thus imply the necessity for draining the surplus to restore bodily balance.[71]

Homeopathy*

Homeopathic remedies, highly controversial among pharmacists as well as skeptics of many denominations, work ostensibly by inciting the immune system and/or enhancing the vital force of the body (whichever terminology one prefers) to regain or increase its capacity to restore balance as pathologies arise. The presumption is that one is sick and symptom-ridden because an inherent therapeutic mechanism has become lethargic or numbed into inactivity by the more elegant design of a disease process. The body also responds to stress or infection by various defensive symptoms.

---

*See *Homeopathy: The Great Riddle,* pp. 31–88; *Planet Medicine: Origins,* pp. 250–251, 287–288, 495–496; *Planet Medicine: Modalities,* pp. 85–86, 590–599; *Embryogenesis,* pp. 610–612; and *Embryos, Galaxies, and Sentient Beings,* pp. 165, 396.

Homeopathy is distinguished by two main features: the doctrine of similars and the potentization of the microdose. The doctrine of similars propounds that a person is most effectively cured by a substance that causes a similar, though not identical, symptom complex to the disease. This is by contrast to allopathy which attempts to cure by counteracting the disease itself, either by giving a remedy with an opposing effect or, in a number of instances, by excising the diseased tissue or intrusion altogether. It is also by contrast with isopathy (immunization and allergology), which uses an altered dose of the *same* substance.

The guiding principle of allopathy is to neutralize or annihilate a toxin or malignancy; the guiding principle of homeopathy is to stimulate the organism to cure itself by a holistic change, encompassing the symptom in its resonance—that is, healing from within.

If an allopathic drug is ingested or surgical procedure enacted, by homeopathic standards the organism has most likely been rendered *more* lethargic and unresponsive, *less* able to defend itself. Though the disease manifestation may be temporarily suppressed and a troublesome symptom vanquished, there is no systemic jolt for the system to revitalize, so it settles into deeper sluggishness. Insofar as the disease must express itself somehow, the symptom will likely recur or be replaced by another symptom, probably more severe, a second-best outlet from a homeostatic standpoint. Since every defect, invader, and pathogen cannot be removed anyway, one by one by one mechanically, the homeopathic strategy is to mobilize the tissues and antibodies to do the work themselves efficiently and holistically, even as they did embryogenically in designing an organism.

A homeopathic similar is meant to be an alternative to the disease, a milder, more recognizable, nonpathological replacement to which the compromised system can respond in an energetic and curative way. The organism has already proven to be incapable of recognizing or reversing the debilitative process in its transparent form; thus, an alias is substituted in order to break systemic fixation and catalyze the needed response.

Homeopathy does not claim to first make a person feel better—in fact, a remedy often increases the vexation of the patient because the cure is working on a parallel track to the disease, fueling its symptoms from the standpoint that the symptoms are not the disease but the organism's response to the disease in attempt to cure itself. Improvement kicks in only after discomfort or pain, as initial hardship often confirms a therapeutic reaction. To exacerbate symptoms within reason is not to enhance the pathology (as it might initially appear during the period of aggravation) but to invigorate the organism. All of this is anathema to allopaths who valorize their opposition to disease and market their trade by swift, mollifying results.

Note how homeopathic language suggests migraine action. A migraine itself may be a form of "homeopathic" cure, thus should not be mitigated allopathically. Conversely, homeopathic potencies can resonate therapeutically with migraines without suppressing their vital or immune responses.

If a physician wanted to treat migraine auras homeopathically, he would prescribe a substance that causes aura-like hallucinations in order to harmonize itself fundamentally with them so that their artifacts no longer have energy to form. An effective remedy might well intensify the scotoma but also make it pass more rapidly. For instance, it might cause it to oscillate at a quicker pulse to the point where its vibration led to thinning and then dissipation. The aura would depart not by slowing down or waning but resonating more swiftly. The potency would in a sense detonate or vaporize it from its own components.*

---

*A remedy with this effect on migrainous flickers in the left eye is *China Arsenicum.*

The proviso here is that, if a migraine is already fundamentally aligned with the organism, it may be more difficult to treat homeopathically than an extrinsic pathology would.

The microdose principle of homeopathy states that the lower the dosage of the medicine given, the more powerful its curative effect and the less toxic its side-effects. This clearly runs against conventional pharmaceutical logic which, except in cases like immunization, does not adopt either a microdose or an isopathic premise.

It might be noted that the original homeopaths did not devise a theoretical premise of minute doses as paradoxically potent and then set out to test it. They began by first applying the ancient idea of similars in a contemporary pharmaceutical context and then incrementally reducing dosages in order to discover how far they could dilute a substance without curtailing its curative effect. There was good reason for this: If one is dispensing medicines that increase fevers and make pains more searing and if (in addition) one is prescribing poisons like arsenic and spider venom, it would be safest to succeed with the lowest active dose.

Because toxic side-effects seemed to decrease with each phase of dilution while therapeutic power concomitantly increased, homeopathy developed uniquely as a science of nanopharmacy, a quantum medicine of extremely tiny doses. However, since it originated and established its paradigm in the late eighteenth and the nineteenth centuries, it did not have the "benefit" of a modern understanding of molecular science, let alone nanoscience or physics, thus identified its effects with unknown principles of pharmaceutical activity, not recognized then and not recognized today by mainstream chemistry and biology. There is no consensus of explanation for the potency of microdoses, even among homeopaths.

The homeopathic microdose is not just a similar substance given in a tiny amount. The medicine must be prepared by a series of reductions of its original mass in a neutral medium (usually sugar water) while being shaken forcefully (succussed) with each reduction. Under these circumstances, homeopaths understand that the molecular properties of the substance are transmuted, intensified, and transferred on a vibrational level to the neutral medium. Then each next dilution and succussion further increase its medicinal force.

Metaphors from quantum physics and the paraphysics of water molecules abound in homeopathy's post-modern lexicon but, except for mentioning the notion that bombarding atoms against one another increases their medical potency, I will leave the reader to peruse these elsewhere (see *Homeopathy: The Great Riddle*, pp. 66–81, for instance). Suffice it to say that natural enzymes in the body in very small amounts approximating homeopathic doses inaugurate powerful, synergistic responses in an organism. Whether molecules cause changes when in the even tinier amounts of some of the higher homeopathic doses (i.e., greater dilutions) is unknown, in part because equipment does not track substances in such miniscule amounts and in part because scientists do not believe that dilutions past a certain level (a level most homeopathic remedies exceed) have any molecules left of the original substance to track, so do not study their "effects." Mysterious meta-molecular vibrations in the absence of material substance are simply not in the repertoire of standard biochemistry or physics.

A microdose, to be effective by homeopathic principles, has to be specifically similar, which means that the succussion has to incite a reaction in the patient very close to the symptoms of the patient's condition. Otherwise, it falls into the background pollution of the body, which already contains a host of other irrelevant and toxic substances that have invaded it from the environment in absurdly higher amounts than most homeopathic remedies. Check any public water supply and one will find many of the worst toxins known to humanity in various dilutions, highly succussed and potentized! Yet, in the same way that an organism responds to the specificity of an enzymatic signal, not only in its metabolism and homeostasis but via the morphogenetic process of developing organs in the womb, so will it ostensibly respond to the meticulously correct homeopathic microdose, *if the underlying etiology of homeopathy is accurate.*

Two interrelated points are worth reemphasizing in relation to the treatment of migraine auras:

One, homeopathy regards the "diseases" of allopathy as symptoms of a real disease which exists solely at an imperceptible systemic and submetabolic level such that it has created an imbalance to which the extant "disease" or symptom is a coping endeavor by the organism, an immune response. The actual, existential core pathology cannot be contacted directly by any remedy, allopathic or homeopathic.

No one knows what a migraine is; they only know its headaches, scotomata, or other characteristic event clusters. An aura is an ineffable, nonspecific substrate with systemic effects. We cannot discern whether, in the economy of the body, it is functioning pathologically in an allopathic sense or therapeutically in a homeopathic sense. We also cannot gauge how much it is a symptomatic channel or how close to the primordium of the disease itself.

Second, homeopathic remedies are prescribed on the basis not of a single symptom or even a set of symptoms but the whole picture of health and disease of the individual. A reputable homeopath would never treat just a person's migraine auras: there is no "aura" remedy; that is, there is no remedy that can cure migraines or auras in everyone. A homeopathic physician will spend hours taking a complete case, compiling an organized list of the patient's symptoms, mental as well as physical: tastes in food, susceptibilities to heat and cold, obsessive thoughts, tics and rashes, etc., and then choose the remedy that comes closest to his or her *entire* organizational pattern. The migraine aura would be only one part of this holistic diagnosis.

Additionally, homeopathy makes no distinction between physical and mental symptoms, since it is treating the disease core, not the symptoms, using the symptoms solely as diagnostic clues to what the core is.

Extensive indices matching remedies with specific symptoms have been compiled over two-plus centuries of homeopathy and are now available as repertories in the form of either bound compendia or computer programs.

Because, as noted, homeopaths select their remedies on the basis of symptom complexes and whole pictures rather than individual symptoms, it would be a bowdlerization to single out any remedies for general treatment of auras here. Below is a sampling of ones that have been successful when auras are part of the individual's picture. All of them emphasize some migraine-aura characteristics over others, and a few symptoms (such as sensitivity to light/noise, scintillation in the field of vision, blind spots, and nausea) show up in many of them; yet the correct "similar" will be validated by other factors such as a patient's food cravings, complexion, emotional qualities, body type, skin blemishes, compulsions, habits, and so on. It is necessary to individualize any migraine remedy on the basis of its non-aura components as well.

My selected homeopathic migraine-aura remedies are annotated with the help of Dana Ullman, a homeopath, and Matthew Wood, an herbalist/homeopath. Do remember (again) that the goal of diagnosis is to arrive at a general picture of an unknowable disease core manifesting through symptoms which differ by individual constitution, so not all the symptoms inventoried occur in all patients for whom the remedy is specified; in fact, few of them converge in any one patient. Rubrics contain *all* symptoms for *all* patients, for conditions minor or severe, chronic or acute, that fit and define the remedy (and disease) in one way or another. Any one person will have, at best, a smattering of elements that suggest the disease's peculiar pattern in them. The art is to draw a picture from a broad constellation of rubrics, not all of which are individually applicable.

Each remedy mentioned below likewise is not the sole treatment for everyone with an itemized symptom:

Carbo Vegetabilis, wood charcoal, is repertorized for scotomata, dimming vision, and circular artifacts around an indistinct visual field. Among its other symptoms are varicose veins, weariness to the point of collapse, extreme flatulence with diarrhea, occipital headaches, cold knees at night, icy coldness of the whole body (even to the point of appearing blue), cold sweats, itchy anus, yellow fever, fainting, burning in the eyes, gangrene, vaso-motor paralysis, stagnant blood, and whooping cough.[72]

Chelidonium Majus, the greater celandine, is related to bloodroot in its homeopathic as well as herbal treatment of migraines. Its migrainous rubrics include right-sided headaches that increase in the forehead and temples with nausea and vomiting; neuralgic pain in the head and face; intense pain in the area of the eyes and eyebrows (also ear pain); photophobia to the point of dread of light; parts of the body (especially the cranium) feeling too small; paralysis of the optic nerve; vertigo; and flickering, sparks, optical illusions, and blind spots in the vision. Among its other symptoms are general sluggishness and lethargy, laziness and lassitude, jaundice (especially of the face), tongue so thickly coated that the margins of the teeth show in it, paroxysms of hollow coughing (particularly in the morning and at 4 P.M.), general mental confusion, tendency toward abstraction and denial, a sensation of wind rushing out of the ears, a stiff neck, pains in shoulders (particularly the inner lower angle of the right shoulder), engorgement of the right lung, golden urine, alternating constipation and diarrhea, bright yellow stools, symptoms improving when lying down, and depression from overcast weather. *Chelidonium* is usually recommended in lower doses (less potentization), which more closely replicates its herbal use.[73]

Coffea Cruda, coffee or caffeine, emphasizes kinesthetic and tactile manifestations such as tingling, neuralgia, things moving too fast, inexplicable pains, but also flickering vision and sparks before the eyes. Other symptoms include mental overactivity, restlessness, talkativeness, grinding of the teeth, a one-sided headache as if from a nail driven into the head, and a reduction of the desire to scratch itches because of their hypersensitivity.[74]

Conium Maculatum, hemlock, is repertorized for both rainbows and dazzling colors in the eye and for double and dimming vision (negative scotomata) as well as photophobia. It is additionally characterized by forgetfulness, hypochondria, indulgence, numbness with pain, vertigo when turning the head, inability to watch moving things or rapid motion without getting a headache, night sweats, swelling of glands, prostate enlargement, an excess of ear wax, and paroxysms of coughing.[75]

Datura Stramonium (also called *Stramonium*), thorn-apple, a narcotic plant in nonhomeopathic doses, is repertorized for sudden loss of vision, chorea, aggravation by bright light, a horror of glistening objects, illusory objects suddenly crawling, hallucinations of ghostlike figures and beasts in the field of vision, and mental confusion such that things are called by the wrong names and a person reaches for articles that are too far away to touch, yet bumps into people and objects nearby. *Stramonium* also elicits fear of being alone, obsessive partying, restlessness, twitching, hydrophobia, an insistence that there are bugs when there aren't (with a desire to catch them), a compulsion for obscenity and swearing, verbosity, a desire to bite things, stumbling over one's own feet, and a craving for vinegar. *Belladonna* is a related remedy with many of the same rubrics.[76]

Ignatia is repertorized for flickering zigzags and a picture of multiple migrainoid elements: hysteria, nausea, spasms, convulsions, mental stress associated with shock and bereavement, long-suppressed and deep grief, throbbing head pain, esophagal formication, a feeling of overall weakness, itchy throat, hiccoughs, waking with a start, and spreading pain from mere light touch.[77]

Kali Biochromicum underscores loss of vision at the beginning of a headache (with the vision returning during the headache), bright spots and colored sparks before the eyes, diplopia, and red hallucinations. Its other rubrics include nausea, the nose feeling too heavy, the tongue leaden and coated, a sensation of something stuck in the esophagus and food lying dormant in the stomach, hoarseness, a metallic cough with white mucus, a craving for beer, a feeling of being unable to empty the urethra of urine, a pain in the coccyx, pustules that won't burst (anywhere on the body), an eruption of vesicles on the scalp, and pain in the anus.[78]

Lycopodium, club moss, repertorizes for fixation from bright light, especially in the evening, e.g. blindness following a flash or glow; also, to a lesser degree, spots and sparks with visual disorientation, selecting the wrong words, and confusion about everyday things. Other *Lycopodium* conditions are excessive appetite even to the point of bloating the stomach, vertigo upon rising from lying down or sleep, melancholia with weeping, bad periods (including revisitations of past ailments) between 4 and 8 P.M., inappropriate amorousness, teeth that hurt when chewing, craving hot and sweet things, symptoms of all sorts moving from right to left and above to below with an emphasis on right-sided ailments, shrunken or frail appearance, hyper-intellectual or pseudo-intellectual posturing, acrid and/or burning urine (sometimes with red sand in it), only the right foot feeling cold, a state of being unrefreshed by sleep, and general crankiness.[79]

Mercurius, mercury, accentuates insect-like distortions before the eyes, a fog blotting out parts of vision, photophobia, and an inability to recognize what one sees. Other rubrics include taste of rotten eggs or saltiness in the mouth, extreme thirst, sweating without ordinary relief (especially at night and in bed), bloody stools, stinging pains, joint inflammation aggravated by heat, milk in the breasts of non-pregnant women and boys, itchy scalp, a sensation that feathers or ice are coming out of the corners of one's ears, slowness to respond to questions, stuttering, scolding quarrelsomeness, toothaches, and bleeding gums.[80]

Natrum Muriaticum, sodium chloride or common salt, stresses dissolution of images while reading or writing, flickers at the beginning of a headache, and fiery zigzags. Other symptoms include weepiness, depression, blisters on the tongue, herpes sores in the mouth and on the arms, bitter tastes, constipation, easy fatigue, facial heat, muddy urine, a feeling as though one's head will explode, morning chills, malaria, a sensation of a cold wind blowing through the head when there is none, and an impression of water trickling in the joints. Though *Nat. mur.* has a reputation for alleviating headaches, it can also make migraine ones temporarily worse from homeopathic aggravation.[81]

Sanguinaria Canadensis, bloodroot, has foggy vision and neuralgia-like aura pains, especially in the head and running down the forehead, often settling over the right eye, and/or crossing the face in all directions from the upper jaw. In addition, it repertorizes for the tongue feeling dry and hot as if it would crack, swollen chest pain, the world moving dizzily around one, dry cough, general lassitude and languor, a feeling of a hard sensation in the stomach, and lameness in the right arm.[82]

Again remember, while these may sound like parodies of actual ailments, they are not ailments are all; they are discrete but nonexclusive elements of a fluid picture; symptoms that overlap, negate one another, and are interchangeable; definitions that are sufficient but not necessary. No one experiences such litanies of symptoms or quirky complaints, and a person embodying the entire picture of any remedy would not be able to get out of bed. The rubrics are guides to selecting a single remedy, the closest similar, over all others; they have no absolute or other relevance.

Acupuncture*

Like homeopathic microdoses, acupuncture needles shoot subtle messages through the neuromusculature, circulatory systems, and tissues. As described above, these pass from their sites of insertion along meridians entering different zones. Most standard doctors are dubious that these metal (or electric) insertions can impart any more than minor symptomatic relief. However, according to the traditional Chinese model, the effect of the needles is to dispatch bioelectrical and morphogenetic signals into tissues, and these have a profound effect in vitalizing the entire system and restoring its elemental harmony. Informal studies have shown that acupuncture is effective in relieving forty percent of migraine headaches, though needle sites and reciprocities differ from patient to patient.

In my earlier discussion of the role of the gallbladder meridian in the etiology of migraines, I took an herbalist's viewpoint, a strategy of following a dominant clinical sign along one trajectory (e.g. a rising liver obstruction) and channeling chemical effects directly into its organ pathway. An experienced acupuncturist would likely not diagnose or treat that way but work in a larger Five Element matrix of symptom, sign, and pattern differentiation, using multiple interdependent qualities of pulses and organ energies as an indi-

---

*See *Planet Medicine: Origins*, pp. 353–359; *Planet Medicine: Modalities*, pp. 96–97; *Embryogenesis*, pp. 605–608, 612–617; and *Embryos, Galaxies, and Sentient Beings*, pp. 281–356.

cation for variable needle placement; he might also prescribe herbs on the same basis. Proper migraine treatment in Chinese medicine is rooted in subtle diagnosis of the interrelationship of meridians and derives from affiliations and interdependencies that are inferred but not seen. Chronic symptoms and declining health will result from treatment of only the symptom-dominant meridian.

For instance, excess ascending heat, a yang condition on the gall-bladder meridian, suggests surplus wind but, since the spleen enhances the liver, the heat and wind may originate more centrally from a yin condition, a weakened spleen with consequent loss of control over its water element, which then sinks. A depleted spleen underwrites liver dominance such that damp heat rising disrupts not just the brain in a linear manner but the heart, mind, and nervous system across a nonlinear network. Healing requires strengthening the spleen by a comprehensive approach, clearing the heat and subduing the wind.[83] Such a strategy honors migraine complexity as we understand it.

Osteopathy and Manual Medicine

Methods of guided palpation and adjustment were incorporated in a general osteopathic tool kit from the dawn of civilization, as different regional traditions of massage, manipulation, and bodywork were cultivated by native craftsmen (and women) and healers across both Old and New Worlds. These have since been syncretized in various Eurasian modes of bodywork and somatic treatments, including light and deep-tissue massage, chiropractic adjustment, and various eclectic modalities of shaking, manipulating, inducing, aligning along fulcra, enhancing fascial vectors, and draining congested areas by light squeezing.* Bodyworkers, like skilled pianists or painters, sense and organize a range of subtle tones or hues.

---

*See *Planet Medicine: Origins,* pp. 147–167.

Palpation improves a number of conditions, not just neuro-muscular ones. All organs can be treated, through cutaneous and subcutaneous layers, intervening fascia, muscles, ribs, and other organs. The bones of the skeleton, especially the spine and cranium, can be manipulated in order to improve the functioning of organs by altering their milieu and range. Palpation can be combined with breath and attention to energize metabolic processes and catalyze static increments in the body-mind.*

Before x-rays, MRIs, ultrasounds, and surgery, physicians *had to* diagnose and heal by the sensitivity of their hands, by the skill of their touch. A manual doctor reads the many pulses, zones of tissue mobility and motility, textures, homunculi, and obstacles in the body and, while deepening his palpation layer by layer, interprets their overall state and attempts to restore or enhance normal ranges of movement and flow. Where there are obstructions and resist-ances, he relieves the force or knot on them and sets them in natu-ral motion again.

Successful palpation must respect the body's innate properties and safeguards. A good osteopath, chiropractor, or physical thera-pist should not force tissues into mechanical function or push them to where he thinks they should ideally go. That would be like try-ing to repair a clock with a hammer—only worse, since the living organism is already a self-repairing clock. Instead the sensitive hands must gauge and weigh signals of balance and imbalance and encour-age them with a pressure no greater than a nickel coin (and often less) to abet their responsiveness and restore their embryogenic rhythms and metabolic potential. This sometimes means guiding

---

*See *Planet Medicine: Modalities,* pp. 141–417 for detailed discussions of the systems mentioned here (as well as the Bates Method, discussed on pp. 77–78). I have gone into depth on the history, practice, and techniques of each modality.

tissues in the direction in which they are stuck, to their furthest range of movement there, and holding them gently at that spot, which excites organ recognition of its trapped situation, causing its increment to counterflow back in the other direction. While taking into account the different, vibrant dynamics of tissue, we might compare this to trying to unscrew a jar lid by rotating it first *in* the direction of tightened threads.*

There are many varieties of bodywork, some more direct, some less; some harder, some lighter; some administered by palpation, some by skeletal adjustment, some by deep massage, some by instructing the client in techniques to reeducate his/her own movement patterns. At one extreme, manual medicine comprises dynamic techniques like Rolfing, which remolds mesodermal tissues, and chiropractic, which reconciles the relation of bones to one another and to organs and circulatory and neural pathways; at the other are the kinds of gentle body exercises taught by Moshe Feldenkrais, F. M. Alexander, and Mabel Todd in the twentieth century as well as other yoga-like and chi-gung systems that work according to similarly meticulous protocols.

Chiropractic adjustments might alleviate a neurocerebral blockage; likewise the exercises and imaging practices of Polarity Therapy or even a martial art like t'ai chi ch'uan could open up skeletal structures, decongest blood flow, and stimulate cerebrospinal circulation, making relevant tissues more supple and cohesive.

Osteopathic, craniosacral, visceral, integrative, and biovalent techniques for working directly on the brain and optic channels by palpating through the eyes, hard palate, and skull go to the heart of the aura-generating system. Osteopathic practitioners and even some neurologists have treated migraine by manual compression in the region of the extracranial arteries, but that is not the only

---

*See *Embryos, Galaxies, and Sentient Beings,* pp. 315–321.

proximal location. Others regard migraine auras as arising specifically from blocks in venous-sinus drainage backing pressure up into the cranium. By palpating within this area and following and releasing the tissues inward, they have gotten occasional relief for both headaches and scotomata.

Practices

Active self-healing techniques include transcendental meditation, zen meditation, and chanting. All of these relax and mobilize tissues and inculcate unique, nonverbal mind-body insights that can serve as direct "homeopathic" improvements of migrainous requisites. There are many modalities in which skilled practitioners can have direct or indirect impact on their own migraines; for instance, one can learn to somatically re-pattern tissues and radiate intentions to sites in the brainstem and visual cortex where the condition likely develops.

Visualization entails imaging the brainwaves, blood vessels, and pathways of the nervous system in their role in forming scotomata in hopes of preemptively reorganizing them. Chi gung, yoga, martial arts (t'ai chi ch'uan, aikido, capoeira, kickboxing, etc.),* and somatic/bodywork (Body-Mind Centering, Continuum, Feldenkrais method, Ideokinesis, Alexander method, etc.)† all teach internal imaging techniques that address auras indirectly by stimulating nerves and muscles and neutralizing stress. In chi gung,‡ one practices motions that massage and lubricate organs and release thera-

---

*See *Planet Medicine: Origins,* pp. 367–374, and *Planet Medicine: Modalities,* pp. 100–107.

†See *Planet Medicine: Modalities,* pp. 182–194, 209–228, 390–415 and *Embryogenesis,* pp. 619–625.

‡See *Planet Medicine: Origins,* pp. 359–367, and *Planet Medicine: Modalities,* pp. 363–374.

peutic energy both in specific viscera and throughout the body. In various bodywork systems, students learn to locate their own subtle organs and regulative homunculi, then direct attention to those that are inert, tense, or stagnant, activating them by coordinated breathing and discrete movements.

The somatic forms mentioned above are among many that teach actions and methods of discriminating and changing physical and mental habits so as to make ordinary activity more natural and free-flowing. Students of Continuum and Body-Mind Centering as well as craniosacral therapy train a capacity to send nonverbal messages in the form of "cell talk," a procedure wherein human thoughts insert intentions in cellular and subcellular activity and steer conscious breathing and focused attention into control centers and matrices of tissues and organelles (or at least into metaphors of these). Regular practice of such skills may alter some of the conditions that underlie auras. The longer the person develops the techniques of these systems, the more conscious the implementation of them becomes and the deeper and more powerful their uncanny effects. An advanced practitioner might well be able to locate his or her own migraine sites and dissolve them, however one understands the concepts implied by those words. Whether one can truly melt aura-generation by meditation, chanting, and other rituals—that is, whether such activities fulfill their own protocols or are more like placebos in arousing the body's natural healing—as long as the desired effect is achieved, the method has succeeded.

It is useful to approach any psychosomatic component in terms of its imaginal elements and engage them even if the encounter turns out to be more semantically than anatomically valid. Per the metabiological logic of life, symbol and event are the same, as both arise from a multidimensional hyperspace that self-propagates once and again into tissues and creatures. It is not a case of talking *to* cells, but energizing human meaning in a biological medium.

Migraine auras are complex, multiform events, unfolding on many levels simultaneously, with a range of co-factors, and advancing through a hierarchy of structures and phenomenologies. Any treatment must take this lineage into account, while also considering migraines' place in the general homeostasis of the systems that they enlist. Insofar as they discharge energy by a benign process and may be an indication of self-regulation in the brain, auras are most effectively addressed by holistic and even paradoxical remedies and therapies. A cautious, respectful approach befits their quantum, existential nature.

Notes*

I. The Nature and Experience of Migraine Auras

1. Janet McKenzie, quoted in "About M.A.G.N.U.M. Awareness Art Gallery," www.migraines.org/about/abouawar.html, p. 3.

2. Derek Robinson, "In the Picture—A Personal View of Migraine," www.migraine-aura.org/EN/In the Picture html, p. 1.

3. Unknown, quoted in "Erich Kæstner," www.migraine-aura.org/EN/Erich·Kaestner.html, p. 1.

4. Sir William Richard Gowers, *Subjective Sensations of Sight and Sound: Abiotrophy, and Other Lectures* (Philadelphia: P. Blakiston's Son & Co., 1904), p. 21.

5. D. Catino, "Ten migraine equivalents," *Headache,* 1965, Vol. 5, pp. 1–11.

6. Caleb Hillier Parry, quoted in Oliver Sacks, *Migraine* (New York: Vintage Books, 1992), pp. 53–54.

7. Hubert Airy, "On a Transient Form of Hemianopsia," *Philosophical Transactions of the Research Society of London,* Vol. 160, pp. 247–270; quoted in Sacks, p. 59.

8. Sir William Richard Gowers, "Subjective Visual Sensations," *Transactions of the Ophthalmological Society of the United Kingdom* 15, 1895, pp. 20–44; quoted in Sacks, p. 55.

9. Gowers, *Subjective Sensations of Sight and Sound: Abiotrophy, and Other Lectures,* p. 36.

---

*I have cited sources and references where I still have them. Other material, especially from among what I collected online, is either no longer available or undocumented there. I will be glad to improve individual references in future printings if readers provide information between editions. Many of the references have been taken intact from the Internet and other secondary sources, so their method of annotation varies, representing what was available in each instance or standardized to the degree possible.

10. Donald M. Pedersen, "Migraine aura without headache," *Journal of Family Practice,* www.findarticles.com/p/articles/mi m0689/is n5 v32/ai 10881173.

11. W. Richards, "The Fortification Illusions of Migraine," *Scientific American* 224, 1971, pp. 88–96.

12. Gowers, *Subjective Sensations of Sight and Sound: Abiotrophy, and Other Lectures,* p. 27.

13. "Migraine Visual Aura Simulation," www.halfbakery.com/idea/ Migraine 20Visual 20Aura 20Stimulation, p. 2.

14. Ibid., pp. 1–2.

15. Ibid., pp. 10, 3–4.

16. Ibid., p. 3.

17. Karl Spencer Lashley, "Patterns of Cerebral Integration Indicated by Scotomas of Migraine," *Archives of Neurological Psychiatry,* Vol. 46, 1941: pp. 332, 331.

18. "Migraine Visual Aura Simulation," pp. 1–2.

19. Gowers, *Subjective Sensations of Sight and Sound: Abiotrophy, and Other Lectures,* p. 25.

20. "Migraine Visual Aura Simulation," p. 2.

21. Ibid., pp. 5–6.

22. www.migraine-aura.org/EN/Kadenza.html, pp. 1–2.

23. "Migraine Visual Aura Simulation," p. 4. [I have punctuated this entry and corrected spelling errors.]

24. "Migraine Art in the Internet," www.migraine-aura.org/EN/Migraine Art in the Internet html, p. 2.

25. Sacks, p. xv.

26. "Migraine Visual Aura Simulation," p. 9.

27. Airy, quoted in Sacks, p. 59.

28. Pedersen, p. 2.

29. "Migraine Visual Aura Simulation," p. 4.

30. Sacks, p. 91.

31. Airy, quoted in Sacks, p. 60.

32. "Migraine Visual Aura Simulation," p. 9.

33. Sacks, p. 56.

34. Robinson, pp. 1–2.

35. Sacks, p. 56.

36. Axel Klee, *A Clinical Study of Migraine with Particular Reference to the Most Severe Cases* (Copenhagen: Munksgaard, 1968); quoted in Sacks, p. 277.

37. Sacks, p. 63.

38. Aretaeus, quoted in Sacks, p. 273.

39. Lashley, p. 335.

40. Ibid.

41. Gowers, *Subjective Sensations of Sight and Sound: Abiotrophy, and Other Lectures*, pp. 23–25.

42. Ibid. pp. 21, 27–28.

43. Sacks, p. 59.

44. Ibid.

45. Ibid.

46. Lashley, pp. 334, 336, 337.

47. Airy, quoted in Sacks, pp. 273–274.

48. Gowers, *Subjective Sensations of Sight and Sound: Abiotrophy, and Other Lectures*, pp. 26–27.

49. Sacks, p. 55

50. Ibid., p. 257.

51. Ibid., p. 56.

52. Gowers, *Subjective Sensations of Sight and Sound: Abiotrophy, and Other Lectures*, pp. 25–26.

53. Ibid., pp. 31–33.

54. Sacks, p. 56.

55. William Burrill, *Welcome to the Fun House*, in *eye weekly*, May 16, 1996; quoted in www.migraine-aura.org/EN/Vincent•van•Gogh.html.

56. Sacks, p. 87.

57. Ibid., p. 56.

58. Ibid., p. 275.

59. Ibid., p. 80.

60. Ibid., p. 279.

61, Axel Klee, quoted in Sacks, p. 75f.

62. "Migraine Visual Aura Simulation," p. 6.

63. Sacks, p. 53.

64. Lashley, pp. 338–339.

65. Robinson, p. 2.

66. Oliver Sacks, *The Man Who Mistook His Wife for a Hat and Other Clinical Tales* (New York: Simon and Schuster/Summit, 1985); Sacks, *Migraine*, p. 76f. [All subsequent footnotes labelled "Sacks" are from *Migraine*.]

67. Sacks, p. 86.

68. Ibid., p. 72.

69. Peter van Vugt, "Migraine and Inspiration: C. L. Dodgson's migraine and Lewis Carroll's literary inspiration: a neurolinguistic perspective," *Humanising Language Teaching*, Year 6, Issue 4, November 2004, p. 3.

70. Robinson, p. 2.

71. C. W. Lippman, "Certain hallucinations peculiar to migraine," *Journal of Nervous and Mental Disease*, Vol. 116, 1952: pp. 346–351.

72. Sacks, p. 85.

73. Ibid., p. 73.

74. Siri Hustvedt, Notes from an Interview, sent by email, August 2004.

75. "Migraine and Music," www.migraine-aura.org/EN/Migraine /Migraine and Music html, p. 4.

76. Sacks, p. 52f.

77. Hildegard of Bingen in Charles Singer, "The Visions of Hildegard of Bingen," *From Magic to Science* (New York: Dover, 1958); quoted by Sacks, p. 301.

78. Emily Dickinson, yourcomputergenius.com/nailincoffin/2005/07/ emily-dickinson.html.

79. Klaus Podoll and Derek Robinson, quoted in "Migraine aura symptoms gave rise to 'Adventures in Wonderland'," Reuters Health, April 20, 1999, reporting on article in *Lancet* 1999; 353: 1366, www.fallindream.blogdrive .com.

80. Deborah Wirtel, "'Alice in Wonderland': A Children's Book or a Migraineur's Diary," headaches.about.com/od/profiles/a/carroll·l.htm.

81. Van Vugt, pp. 3–4.

82. Wirtel, op. cit.

83. This list was compiled from van Vugt and Wirtel.

84. Van Vugt, p. 3.

85. Podoll and Robinson; see also www.migraine-aura.orgn/EN/Lewis·

Carroll.html for version of the discussion that includes Carroll's journal notes and illustrations.

86. www.migraine-aura.org/EN/Vincent van Gogh. html.

87. www.ibiblio.org/wm/paint/auth/seurat/baignade and www.gbcnv.edu/
•techdesk/Diana/works.html.

88. Razia Iqbal, "Migraine theory on Picasso paintings," news.bbc.uk/l/hi/
world/europe/909914.stm, p. 2.

89. "The Migraine Art Competitions," www.migraine-aura.org/EN/The Migraine Art Competitions.html, pp. 1–2.

91. Ibid., pp. 3–4.

91. Deborah Hartzman, Newsgroups: alt.support.headaches.migraine, March 16, 1995; quoted in "Migraine Art Exhibitions," www.migraine-aura.org/EN/Migraine Art Exhibitions.html, p. 2.

92. Barbara Ronda's migrainepage on-line journal, 1996 Journal Entries, July 1996 (4/5); quoted in "Migraine Art Exhibitions," www.migraine-aura.org/EN/Migraine Art Exhibitions.html, p. 2.

93. "Migraine Art in the Internet," www.migraine-aura.org/EN/Migraine Art in the Internet.html, p. 1.

94. "Migraine and Music," www.migraine-aura.org/EN/Migraine and Music.html, pp. 1–4.

95. Ibid., p. 3.

96. Ibid.

97. Ibid.

98. Ibid., p. 4.

99. "Art brut and Migraine Art," www.migraine-aura.org/EN/Georgia O'Keeffe.html.

100. Joan Didion, "In Bed," sunsite.wits.ac.za/holistic/didion.htm, pp. 1–2; from *The White Album* (New York: Noonday Press, 1990).

101. Pedersen, p. 1.

102. Timothy C. Hain, "Migraine Headache," www.dizziness-and-balance.com/disorders/central/migraine/MIGRAIN6.html, August 2005, p. 1.

103. W. C. Alvarez, "The Migraine Scotoma as Studied in 618 Persons," *American Journal of Ophthalmology*, Vol. 49, 1960, p. 489; quoted in Sacks, p. 88.

104. Ibid.

105. Sacks, p. 88f.

106. "Migraine Visual Aura Simulation," p. 6. [I have punctuated this entry and corrected spelling errors.]

107. C. P. Schreiber and others, "Prevalence of migraine in patients with a history of self-reported or physician-diagnosed 'Sinus' headache," *Archives of Internal Medicine,* Vol. 164, 2004, pp. 1769–1772.

108. Sacks, p. 121.

109. Y. River, T. Ben Hur, and I. Steiner, "Reversal-of-vision metamor-phopsia: clinical and anatomical characteristics," *Archives of Neurology,* Vol. 55, #10, October 1998: pp. 1285–1286.

110. Marvin Minsky, "Migraine and Literature," www.migraine-aura.org/EN/Marvin Minsky.html, pp. 1–2.

111. Sacks, p. 136.

112. Ibid., pp. 83, 87.

113. Robinson, p. 1.

114. Sacks, pp. 63–64.

115. Ibid., p. 85.

116. Ibid., p. 86.

117. Ibid., p. 141.

118. Ibid., p. 160.

119. Ibid., pp. 151–152.

120. Ibid., p. 161.

121. "Migraine Visual Aura Simulation," p. 11.

122. Sacks, p. 169.

123. Ibid., pp. 155–160.

124. "Migraine Visual Aura Simulation," p. 4.

125. Sacks, p. 31.

126. Edward Living, quoted in Sacks, p. 31.

127. Sacks, p. 84.

128. Hildegard of Bingen, quoted in Sacks, p. 301.

129. Sacks, p. 83.

130. Ibid., p. 97.

131. Hustvedt, op. cit.

132. Fyodor Dostoyevsky, quoted in Sacks, p. 301.

133. Sacks, p. 76f.

134. W. Gooddy, quoted in Sacks, p. 139.

135. Sacks, p. 98.

136. Ibid., pp. 94–95.

137. Ibid., p. 95.

138. Siri Hustvedt, *The Blindfold: A Novel* (New York: Henry Holt and Company/Picador, 1992), pp. 67–68.

139. Ibid., p. 93.

II. The Biology of Migraine Auras

1. Sacks, p. 201.

2. Lashley, p. 339.

3. Sacks, p. 32.

4. Ibid., p. 28.

5. Ibid., pp. 195–197, 264.

6. Ibid., pp. 258–259.

7. References for this list, up to the last four entries, are: Sacks, pp. 178–183, 187; Timothy C. Hain, "Migraine Headache," www.dizziness-and-balance.com/disorders/central/migraine/MIGRAIN6.html, August 2005, pp. 1–2; and Donald M. Pedersen, "Migraine aura without headache," *Journal of Family Practice*, www.findarticles.com/p/articles/mi m0689/is n5 v32/ai 10881173, pp. 2–3.

8. Manuel Sanchez-del-Rio, "Migraine aura: new information on underlying mechanisms," *Current Opinions in Neurology*, Vol. 17, #3, June 2004.

9. A. Gasbarrini, "Beneficial effects of *Helicobacter pylori* eradication on migraine," *Hepatogastroenterology*, Vol. 45, 1998: pp. 765–770.

10. Ben Harder, "Against the Migraine: A procedure's serendipitous success hints that some migraines start in the heart," www.sciencenews.org/articles/20050219/bob8.asp, February 19, 2005, Vol. 167, #8, pp. 119–124.

11. Sacks, p. 274.

12. J. F. W. Herschel, quoted in Sacks, p. 274.

13. Gowers, *Subjective Sensations of Sight and Sound: Abiotrophy, and Other Lectures*, p. 20.

14. Lashley, p. 338.

15. Sacks, p. 288.

16. Ibid.

17. Ibid., p. 188.

18. Pedersen, p. 3.

19. Sacks, p. 258.

20. Y. River, T. Ben Hur, and I. Steiner, "Reversal-of-vision metamorphopsia: clinical and anatomical characteristics," *Archives of Neurology*, Vol. 55, #10, October 1998: pp. 1–2.

21. Hain, p. 2.

22. D. A. Marcus, *Expert Opinions in Pharmacology*, Vol. 4, #9, September 2003: p. 1609; quoted in www.ncbi.nlm.nih.gov/entrez/query/fcgi?cmd.

23. Sacks, p. 200.

24. Ibid., p. 199.

25. Ibid., p. 190.

26. Ibid., p. 289.

27. Ibid., pp. 195–196.

28. Ibid., p. 196.

29. Ibid., p. 260.

30. M. Sanchez-del-Rio, p. 289.

31. Sacks, pp. 34–35.

32. Ibid., p. 45.

33. Ibid., p. 208.

34. Gowers, *Subjective Sensations of Sight and Sound: Abiotrophy, and Other Lectures*, p. 33.

35. Sacks, p. 45.

36. "Mixed up in space: Humans can become confused and disorganized—and even a little queasy—in an alien world where up and down have no meaning," science.nasa.gov/headlines/y2001/ast07aug•1.html.

37. Jeronimo Cardano, quoted Sacks, pp. 302–303.

38. Swami Vishnu-devananda, *Meditation and Mantras* (New York: Om Lotus Publishing, 1978), p. 240.

39. Karma Chagmé, *Naked Awareness* (Ithaca, New York: Snow Lion Publications, 2000), pp. 160–178.

40. I am grateful to Michael Tweed, editor for Rangjung Yeshe Publications of Nepal, for helping to compose some of this section.

41. Sacks, pp. 32–33.

42. Charles Sherrington, quoted in Sacks, p. 297.

43. Sacks, p. 290.

44. Ilya Prigogine, quoted in Sacks, p. 286 (indirect quote).

45. Ibid., p. 291f.

46. Sacks, p. 291.

47. James Gleick, *Chaos: Making a New Science* (New York: Viking Penguin, 1987), pp. 122–124 *et seq.*, 209–211 *et seq.*

48. Ibid., pp. 137–140 *et seq.*

49. Ibid., pp. 60–79, 83–86.

50. Ibid., pp. 53–56.

51. J. F. W. Herschel, quoted in Sacks, p. 274.

52. Gleick, pp. 94–110.

53. Sacks, p. 279.

54. Ibid.

55. Ibid, p. 294.

56. Ibid., p. 292.

57. Ibid., pp. 291–292.

58. J. Allan Hobson and Hellmut Wohl, *From Angels to Neurones: Art and The New Science of Dreaming* (Fidenza, Italy: Mattioli 1885 spa, 2005), pp. 37–39, 53–55. I'd like to thank Stephen Chorover of the Department of Brain and Cognitive Sciences, Massachusetts Institute of Technology, for providing me with the insight underlying this section and lending me the above-mentioned book, a signed copy from the first author to him, to help write it.

III. The Treatment of Migraine Auras

1. Donald M. Pedersen, "Migraine aura without headache," *Journal of Family Practice,* www.findarticles.com/p/articles/mi m0689/is n5 v32/ai 10881173, p. 4. Sacks, pp. 52–53, 89–92.

2. Pedersen, pp. 3–4.

3. Timothy C. Hain, "Migraine Headache," www.dizziness-and-balance .com/disorders/central/migraine/MIGRAIN6.html, August 2005, p. 2; Pedersen, pp. 4–5.

4. "The Saint, the King's Grandson, the Poet, and the Victorian Writer: Instances of MS When the Disease Did Not Have a Name," *International Journal of MS Care,* Vol. 3, Issue 2, June 2001, p. 1 *et seq.*

5. Pedersen, p. 5.

6. Hain, p. 2.

7. Ibid.

8. Ibid.

9. Ibid.

10. Sacks, p. 252.

11. Ibid.

12. Ben Harder, "Against the Migraine: A procedure's serendipitous success hints that some migraines start in the heart," www.sciencenews.org/articles/20050219/bob8.asp, February 19, 2005, Vol. 167, #8, pp. 119–124.

13. Sacks, pp. 42–43.

14. Ibid., pp. 253–254.

15. Madhuleema Chaliha, "The Beauty of Having a Migraine," mail-archive.com/assm@pikespeak.uccs.edu.msg04629.html, 28 June, 2003: 41:42–0700.

16. Siri Hustvedt, Notes from an Interview, sent by email, August 2004.

17. Sacks, p. 254.

18. Alexander Mauskop, M.D., and Barry Fox, Ph.D., *What Your Doctor May Not Tell You About Migraines* (New York: Time Warner, 2001); Sue Dyson, *Migraines: A Natural Approach* (Berkeley, California: Ulysses Press, 2002); Sacks.

19. Ibid.

20. Hain, p. 11.

21. Ibid.

22. Hain, p. 3.

23. Hain, p. 3; Mauskop and Fox; Dyson; Sacks.

24. I am grateful to Robert Zeiger, an acupuncturist, herbalist, and former pharmacist, for help with this section.

25. Hain, pp. 9–10.

26. Ibid., p. 7.

27. Sacks, p. 263.

28. Joan Didion, "In Bed," sunsite.wits.ac.za/holistic/didion.htm, pp. 1–2; from *The White Album* (New York: Noonday Press, 1990).

29. Hain, pp. 6–7.

30. Ibid., pp. 3–4, 6–7.

31. Ibid., pp. 6–7, 12.

32. Ibid., p. 5.

33. Ibid., pp. 6–9.

34. Hustvedt, Notes from an Interview, sent by email, August 2004.

35. Hain, pp. 4–5.

36. Ibid., p. 5.

37. Ibid., p. 4.

38. Ibid., p. 5.

39. Ibid., p. 4.

40. Ibid., p. 5.

41. Ibid., pp. 4–6.

42. Sacks, p. 261.

43. Hain, p. 3.

44. Ibid., pp. 3, 5.

45. Ibid.

46. A. M. Larson *et al.,* "Acetaminophen-induced acute liver failure: Results of a United States multicenter prospective study," *Hepatology,* Vol. 42, #6, 2005, pp. 1364–1372.

47. Hain, pp. 7–8.

48. Ibid., p. 4.

49. Ibid., pp. 9–10.

50. Ibid., pp. 3, 4.

51. Ibid., p. 6.

52. Nicolas Culpepper, *Complete Herbal,* quoted in M. L. Tyler, *Homoeopathic Drug Pictures* (Bradford, England: Health Sciences Press, 1942), p. 245.

53. Matthew Wood, *The Book of Herbal Wisdom: Using Plants as Medicines* (Berkeley, California: North Atlantic Books, 1997), pp. 211–217.

54. Hain, p. 14.

55. Ibid.

56. Ibid.

57. Jeanne Rose, *The Aromatherapy Book: Applications and Inhalations* (Berkeley, California: North Atlantic Books, 1992), p. 163.

58. Dana Ullman, email written in December 2005, and Matthew Wood, phone conversation, December 2005.

59. Wood, pp. 165–177.

60. Ibid., pp. 219–224.

61. This remedy is provided by Marcey Shapiro, M.D., 2005.

62. Wood, pp. 85–111.

63. Ibid., pp. 499–508.

64. Ibid., pp. 317–321.

65. Hain, p. 9.

66. Ibid.

67. Dana Ullman, email written in December 2005, also directing me to his website www.homeopathic.com/Merchant2/merchant.mvc.

68. Mauskop and Fox, www.twbookmark.com/books/16/0446678260, pp. 6–9.

69. Rose, pp. 69, 88, 107–109, 114, 124–125, 132–133, 164.

70. Hain, p. 9.

71. Sacks, p. 238.

72. James Tyler Kent, *Kent's Repertory with Word Index: Sides of the Body and Drug Affinities—Relationship of Remedies* (New Delhi: B. Jain Publishers Pvt. Ltd., 1905), pp. 271–285; M. L. Tyler, *Homoeopathic Drug Pictures* (Bradford, England: Health Sciences Press, 1942), pp. 206–213.

73. Kent, pp. 271–285; Tyler, pp. 244–251.

74. Kent, pp. 271–285; Tyler, pp. 300–301.

75. Kent, pp. 271–285; Tyler, pp. 320–331.

76. Kent, pp. 271–285; Tyler, pp. 116–126, 768–780.

77. Kent, pp. 271–285; Tyler, pp. 424–431.

78. Kent, pp. 271–285; Tyler, pp. 453–461.

79. Kent, pp. 271–285; Tyler, pp. 513–522.

80. Kent, pp. 271–285; Tyler, pp. 536–545.

81. Kent, pp. 271–285; Tyler, pp. 567–574.

82. Kent, pp. 271–285; Tyler, pp. 728–731.

83. I am grateful to Robert Zeiger, an acupuncturist and herbalist, for help with the last two paragraphs of this section.

Index

Page numbers in *italics* indicate illustrations. Page numbers appended with "n" indicate a footnote (e.g. 102n)

A graduate of Amherst College, Richard Grossinger received a Ph.D. in anthropology from the University of Michigan, writing an ethnography of fishing in Maine. He is the author of many books, including *Planet Medicine; The Night Sky; Embryogenesis: Species, Gender, and Identity; Embryos, Galaxies, and Sentient Beings: How the Universe Makes Life; Homeopathy: The Great Riddle;* and *On the Integration of Nature: Post-9/11 Biopolitical Notes.* He and his wife Lindy Hough are the founding publishers of North Atlantic Books in Berkeley, California.